'This practical and exciting activity manual is a welcome addition to the literature. Robin's clear instructions and astute choice of activities will ensure that care workers have the means to make real positive enhancements to the lives of older people in their care.'

– Danny Walsh, Senior Lecturer, University of Lincoln, UK

'As modern technology and medicine increases life span and the potential for social isolation, Dynes' *Positive Communication*, published by Jessica Kingsley, offers a timely, creative and motivational lifeline. Designed for group facilitators and older adults, it addresses important communication and well-being issues in helpful and practical ways. Highly recommended.'

– Marylyn Cropley, www.freeplay.1me.net

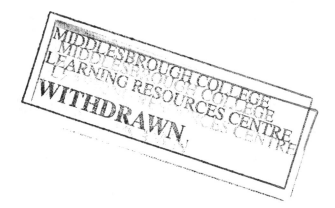

POSITIVE
COMMUNICATION

of related interest

Life Story Work with People with Dementia
Ordinary Lives, Extraordinary People
Edited by Polly Kaiser and Ruth Eley
ISBN 978 1 84905 505 5
eISBN 978 0 85700 914 2

A Creative Toolkit for Communication in Dementia Care
Karrie Marshall
ISBN 978 1 84905 694 6
eISBN 978 1 78450 206 5

Activities for Older People in Care Homes
A Handbook for Successful Activity Planning
Sarah Crockett
ISBN 978 1 84905 429 4
eISBN 978 0 85700 839 8

How to Make Your Care Home Fun
Simple Activities for People of All Abilities
Kenneth Agar
ISBN 978 1 84310 952 5
eISBN 978 1 84642 881 4

The Activity Year Book
A Week by Week Guide for Use in Elderly Day and Residential Care
Anni Bowden and Nancy Lewthwaite
ISBN 978 1 84310 963 1
eISBN 978 1 84642 889 0

POSITIVE
COMMUNICATION

ACTIVITIES TO REDUCE ISOLATION AND IMPROVE THE WELLBEING OF OLDER ADULTS

ROBIN DYNES

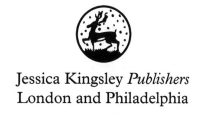

Jessica Kingsley *Publishers*
London and Philadelphia

First published in 2017
by Jessica Kingsley Publishers
73 Collier Street
London N1 9BE, UK
and
400 Market Street, Suite 400
Philadelphia, PA 19106, USA

www.jkp.com

Library of Congress Cataloging in Publication Data
Title: Positive communication : activities to improve the wellbeing of older
   adults / Robin Dynes.
Description: London ; Philadelphia : Jessica Kingsley Publishers, 2017.
Identifiers: LCCN 2016058444 (print) | LCCN 2017016076 (ebook) | ISBN
   9781784504496 (ebook) | ISBN 9781785921810 (alk. paper)
Subjects: LCSH: Older people--Communication. | Interpersonal
   communication--Problems, exercises, etc. | Nursing homes--Activity
   programs.
Classification: LCC BF724.85.I57 (ebook) | LCC BF724.85.I57 D96 2017 (print)
   | DDC 155.67/19--dc23

British Library Cataloguing in Publication Data
A CIP catalogue record for this book is available from the British Library

ISBN 978 1 78592 181 0
eISBN 978 1 78450 449 6

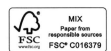
MIX
Paper from
responsible sources
FSC® C016379

Printed and bound in Great Britain

All resources marked with a ★ can be downloaded at www.jkp.com/voucher
using the code DYNESCOMMUNICATION

CONTENTS

THANKS AND ACKNOWLEDGEMENTS

My thanks go to all my friends and colleagues with whom I have been involved while facilitating groups over the past 30 or so years and who have generously shared their knowledge, games and adaptations of activities. It has been a joy to work with you all. As always, I am grateful to my wife, Barbara, for her support and for casting her editorial eye over the text of this book.

INTRODUCTION

ABOUT THIS BOOK

As people grow older, many things conspire against individuals, which influence how they communicate and relate to others. The list is long. Confidence and self-esteem may be eroded by hearing or sight loss. They are affected by illness or physical inability to get about. Family members and friends are lost through death or separation. Having to move to more suitable or manageable accommodation and changes to personal relationships destroy old communication patterns and links. They have to adapt to social and cultural changes which progress as fast as technological changes. Social expectations, shaped by peers and the events and experiences of their time, are out of tune with modern attitudes and the support services are provided by younger people with a different outlook on life.

On top of all this, a youth-orientated society often makes them feel unimportant, inadequate, isolated and obsolete. Day centres, residential homes and nursing homes designed to support them bring them into contact with others who have vastly different interests and backgrounds – ethnic, religious, social and economic. They often see staff as providers of services, not as individuals. Frequently, communication is reduced to making demands or complaining.

Older adults who maintain their communication skills and continue to interact socially maintain a more positive view about themselves and are more adept at facing these challenges. They are more able to cope with changes, communicate their feelings, express opinions and wishes and continue to contribute to society. They are more likely to maintain good physical and emotional wellbeing and maintain their sense of control and achievement in the modern world.

This book provides a range of activities to aid activity organisers help older people maintain their life skills and improve their wellbeing. This might be in residential homes, drop-in or day centres, hospices, clubs for the elderly, hospitals, nursing homes or support situations at home with carers.

USING THE ACTIVITIES

The activities are structured to make it easy to understand their purpose, the materials you will need and what to do. Some additional comments are provided to give further suggestions or tips. Although they have been divided into sections, for ease of finding an activity to suit your purpose, you will find that many would easily fit under more than one heading.

The activities vary in the length of time they will require to complete them. Some can be completed in around 10–15 minutes or so, depending on the number of people in the group and their abilities. Others will take one or more sessions. Be sure to make changes to the topics provided to include social and cultural issues and individual needs. Also, feel free to adapt activities to your personal style and group member goals.

MAKING ALLOWANCES FOR DIFFERENT ABILITIES

You will need to adjust the activities to make allowances for different mental and physical abilities. With a little thought, most of the activities can be made simpler or more challenging. Some group members may need assistance to complete the handouts because of sight impairment or physical difficulties, or they lack the ability to read or write. Even in today's enlightened age many older people and, too frequently, younger people are reluctant, or refuse, to take part in group activities because of problems with reading or writing. This can often be resolved by getting people to work in small groups or pairs – making sure anyone with difficulties is paired with a staff member or someone who is sensitive to their needs. If you know your group members well you'll be aware of what support or equipment they might need in order to feel comfortable when completing any activity.

SETTING THE TONE

Project enthusiasm, fun and enjoyment into the activities. Build a sense of trust and cohesion in the group and ensure that participants have an agreement about confidentiality regarding any personal disclosures. This will go a long way towards helping individuals to feel safe as they take part and to enter into the spirit of the activity without fear.

An enthusiastic, sincere and caring approach is infectious. If you, the group leader, enjoy the activities the magic will hopefully work for everyone.

PARTICIPANTS

It is anticipated that the activities will be used in a wide variety of settings. This means a wide range of abilities, ages, backgrounds and cultures. Some will be mixed, others not. You will need to take this into account when choosing activities and adapt them to suit.

THE FACILITATOR

Everyone develops their own style and methods for making their group successful. An activity that works well for one person with a particular group will not necessarily be successful for someone else running another group. Indeed, you may find that using the same activity with the same group on different days achieves a different response. Here are a few points to keep in mind:

- Think through what you are going to do and plan the activities.

- Choose activities which you can adapt and make suitable to the size of the group, space available and the resources and support you can provide. Take into account the needs of participants and their ability to concentrate and interact with each other. The activity or session should be challenging but not too long – adjust it accordingly.

- Plan assistance for those who need support.

- Make sure you are familiar with the activity and can explain what has to be done. Do any preparation well in advance so you don't have to keep people waiting.

- Introduce the activity in a manner which sets the tone and explains why it is being used.

- Be prepared to repeat and clarify instructions – several times if necessary – for those who have not heard or understood.

- Be liberal with praise and encouragement.

- Respect participants' rights not to share feelings, emotions and private information.

- Maintain a sense of humour. It will frequently save the day.

- At the end of the activity or session summarise what has been achieved and discuss as necessary. Show interest in whether or not people have enjoyed it or found it useful. Feedback information will be useful for when you next use the activity.

KEEPING IT SAFE

It is essential that individuals feel safe, emotionally and physically. Having some agreed group rules which include confidentiality will help. Also, caution needs to be exercised when discussing difficult topics or stimulating personal experiences. A wide variety of emotions can be triggered, ranging from sadness to happiness, anger to joy, and grief to elation. What support can you call on if anyone becomes upset or is having a bad day and needs to leave the group? If any issues surface that need professional input do you have referral routes in place? Think through your risk assessment plan for the group. Make sure you have taken emotional as well as physical safety elements into account.

Because of their special needs, does a particular participant require their own assessment? This might be due, for example, to sight impairment, panic attacks, medical conditions or behavioural difficulties. Your plan should detail action to be taken to reduce any risk – emotional or physical – to that person or other people to an acceptable level. The setting in which you are working should have a policy on these matters. Ensure you comply with it.

COPING WITH POSSIBLE PROBLEMS

Problems crop up in most groups from time to time. You may not always be able to prevent them but you will have to deal with them when they occur. Here are a few common problems, with possible solutions.

Negative and destructive remarks

Have a few basic ground rules with group members, agreeing on what is acceptable and not acceptable within the context of the group. Make sure that this includes what is acceptable behaviour.

Group members want you to provide all the answers to issues being discussed

Redirect comments or questions back to the group. Ask something like: 'What do other group members feel about this?' or 'Some of you have had similar experiences – how did you deal with it?' Alternatively, write the question or statement on a flipchart and brainstorm possible solutions with the group.

Individuals feel uncomfortable

Interacting and communicating with other people involves feelings and emotions – this opens up all sorts of possibilities. However, it remains the participant's choice whether or not to express them. Accept what they feel they can give.

With some of the activities, issues that are uncomfortable for participants may surface. Take care not to force anyone further than they want to go. If a person shows signs of agitation or discomfort with particular issues, accept their decision on how far they want to participate. They can listen to what others have to say without contributing themselves.

Dealing with emotion

Strong emotional responses may be provoked in individuals by an activity. This may be activated by reflecting on past experiences that trigger painful memories. Different situations will need different responses. Here are a few suggestions:

- Reassure the person it is OK to show emotion in the group.

- Create a coffee break to deal with the situation or break tension.

- If necessary have a co-worker take the person out of the group for a cup of coffee or a chat. Do make sure, though, that someone comes back to reassure the other group members that everything is OK or brings the person back.

- Acknowledge with the group what has happened and discuss strategies for them to support anyone who becomes upset in the future. Ask members how they would like to be treated when they feel upset. People differ: one participant might like to be given a few minutes on their own to compose themselves; another person might like to be comforted by someone.

- Have a follow-up chat with the person after the activity. There may be an issue that requires following through by a specialist professional. A general group is not a suitable forum in which to handle extremely sensitive issues such as abuse, self-harm, thoughts of suicide or domestic violence.

When no one wants to talk

Sometimes when approaching difficult topics there can be a reluctance to talk. Everyone feels uneasy and there is an anxious atmosphere. Individuals may be reluctant to speak out. It may be that not enough trust has been developed within the group for members to handle it. If this occurs, or if the activity gets 'stuck' for any reason, try the following:

- Talk about what you think is wrong. Start by saying something like: 'I think some of you are feeling a bit uncomfortable because…' Stating the problem and talking about it often helps people to broach the subject and feel easier.

- Ask members what they think is wrong. You can do this directly to everyone. Or divide them into small groups of three or four people to discuss what is wrong and then feed back to all participants.

- Broach the topic by disclosing how you are feeling, for example: 'I feel that the activity is not going very well. Can you help me with this so we can put it right?' If you encourage people to bring the problem out into the open it can then be worked on.

- Go back to safe topics on a less personal level until more trust has been gained and people feel more comfortable.

One person dominates discussions

Thank the dominant person for their view and ask someone else to comment. Alternatively, have a ground rule that each person is given a limited time to state their views. Or, to prevent anyone becoming dominant, you can invite participants to work in subgroups or pairs. If the behaviour persists, talk to the person away from the group. Focus on the behaviour, not the person. Say something like: 'You are making a valuable contribution to the group but you are not giving other people the opportunity to express their views.'

FINALLY

It is hoped that this book will spark your imagination for other activities to provide safe frameworks within which people can communicate positively, reveal their feelings and wishes for the future, cope with difficult situations, meet their needs, maintain their physical and spiritual wellbeing, enjoy themselves and enhance the quality of their lives. You will laugh a lot and shed some tears in the process of enabling this to happen. That is life! I wish you success in your goal.

All resources marked with a ★ can be downloaded at www.jkp.com/voucher
using the code DYNESCOMMUNICATION

IDENTIFYING STRENGTHS, INTERESTS, HOPES AND DREAMS

ACTIVITIES TO MAINTAIN A POSITIVE OUTLOOK

THE BENEFITS OF STAYING ACTIVE

PURPOSE

To explore the benefits of staying active both mentally and physically.

WHAT YOU'LL NEED

A whiteboard or flipchart and markers.

WHAT TO DO

Ask group members what sorts of activities they have done in the past – both active and creative – to relax, as a pastime or for enjoyment. Write the comments on a whiteboard or flipchart. Examples are:

- » Crosswords
- » Drawing
- » Going for walks
- » Listening to music
- » Gardening
- » Decorating
- » Flower arranging
- » Playing football

When a lengthy list has been completed, ask them what benefits they derived from these activities. Write these on the board or chart. They might include:

- » Helped me relax
- » Stimulated me
- » Boosted my self-esteem
- » Helped me socialise with other people
- » Kept my brain sharp
- » Enabled me to keep fit
- » Helped me lose weight

» Broke the boredom

» Slept better

» Stayed more mobile and independent

» Walking always helped me think things through

» Exercise always improved my mood, got rid of tension and made me feel better

» Provided companionship

When this list is complete, ask: 'What happens if you don't do very much?' Write these comments on the board or flipchart. They may include:

» Getting depressed or low in mood

» Your mind stops working as well as it should

» You don't feel good about yourself

» You are less able to focus and concentrate

Now ask: 'If you keep active mentally and physically now, what will be the result?' Responses might include:

» Less likely to get depressed

» Feel better

» Be able to focus and concentrate better

» Less likely to have memory problems

» Be able to sleep better

» Feel more relaxed

» Stay independent for longer

End the activity by stating that even a small change – introducing a bit more physical and creative activity – in a daily routine can boost morale, provide a sense of achievement and improve how people feel about themselves. Ask participants, in turn, to state one thing they could do to stay more active physically or mentally.

COMMENT

If working with a large group, instead of writing on a board or flipchart, break the group into two or more subgroups and give out large sheets of paper with markers with the headings 'Active and creative activities I have done in the past', 'Benefits derived from these activities', 'What happens if I don't do very much' and 'The result if I keep mentally and physically active'. Each subgroup discusses and completes their charts. When complete, bring the group back together and have each subgroup present their findings.

Instead of asking participants to state one thing they could do to stay more active physically and mentally, you could use this activity in conjunction with the activity 'Making Changes to Stay Active', which provides a method to work with people to introduce small changes.

MAKING CHANGES TO STAY ACTIVE

PURPOSE

To identify current hobbies, interests and activities participants would like to try in the future to keep mentally and physically active.

WHAT YOU'LL NEED

A whiteboard or flipchart and marker, copies of the handout 'Making Changes to Stay Active' and pens.

WHAT TO DO

If you have not done 'The Benefits of Staying Active' activity, start by inviting group members to call out all types of active and creative activities that they have enjoyed in the past or might like to do now. Write the suggestions on a whiteboard or flipchart.

Once you have a long list of activities, give out the handout 'Making Changes to Stay Active'. Ask participants to fill it in one step at a time. After each step, stop and discuss any problems or issues that have arisen. After the action plan has been completed, invite group members, one at a time, to read out what they intend to do.

COMMENT

After completing Step One, some participants may already have quite a full programme of activities, but they might like to substitute some time doing something inactive, such as watching TV or reading, for a more active activity such as dancing or playing skittles, or just something different from what they normally do. When they have decided on a new activity, they will be able to see from Step One where any extra or new activity might fit in. Some problem solving might also need to take place when people are unable to see how they can be enabled to do something they want to do. Also, watch out for anyone trying to take on too much – one or two new activities at a time will be enough, especially if the person is taking part in them more than once a week.

HANDOUT: MAKING CHANGES TO STAY ACTIVE

Step 1: Active and creative activities I do now

Day	Morning	Afternoon	Evening
Sunday			
Monday			
Tuesday			
Wednesday			
Thursday			
Friday			
Saturday			

Step 2: Active and creative things I would like to do involving:

Art (Drawing, colouring, collage, card-making, etc.)	
Words (Creative writing, drama, writing poetry, reading, word puzzles, etc.)	
Music (Dancing, singing, playing music, music appreciation, etc.)	
Craft (Flower arranging, glass painting, jewellery-making, card-making, etc.)	
Cooking (Baking, making jam, etc.)	
Fun and relaxation (Visiting art galleries or garden centres, walking, Yoga, swimming, table tennis, indoor skittles, etc.)	
Other (Gardening, fishing, woodwork, photography, pottery, etc.)	

Step 3: Action plan

Activities I choose to do are:	
I will start doing this on:	
What I need to do to prepare for this is:	

CREATING A BLISS LIST

PURPOSE

To identify enjoyable activities to boost energy when feeling low, stay motivated, fight boredom and manage stress.

WHAT YOU'LL NEED

Pens and paper.

WHAT TO DO

Explain to group members that we can go for days, weeks or months without doing any of the simple things that make us feel good. One way to correct this is to create a list of as many things and activities as possible that make us feel good. These might include simple things like:

» Listening to favourite music

» Writing a poem

» A short walk in the garden or park

» Tea and a chat with a friend

» A visit to the local shopping centre

» Playing a game of Monopoly

» A drive in the country

» A manicure

» A foot massage

» Seeing a grandchild

» Eating chocolate

Give out pens and paper and ask each person to create a list of things that make them feel good – at least ten items. When completed, invite them to share some of the things on their lists. Then ask participants how they are going to make sure that items on their list are included in their weekly or monthly schedules.

COMMENT

Bliss lists should be typed out and posted in places that will ensure they are viewed regularly. You can include in the activity time for each person to make their very own 'bliss list board' on which they can pin or attach notes or pictures showing the things which give them pleasure. Also, point out that it is important that lists need to be kept up-to-date. New things can be tried and added.

HAVING A GOAL

PURPOSE

To motivate people and give an energy boost when they are feeling low.

WHAT YOU'LL NEED

Copies of the handout 'Having a Goal' and pens.

WHAT TO DO

Give out the handout 'Having a Goal' and have participants spend about fifteen minutes completing the form. Explain that the idea is to write down increasingly more ambitious goals in their personal, social and work/leisure areas of life. They should aim for two or three goals in each area. Examples you can give might be:

	Immediate	Reasonable	Wild
Personal	Tidy my room	Buy a new skirt and top	Visit my son in Turkey
Social	Ring my friend Janet	Invite a couple of friends out for lunch	Have a huge family get-together on my 80th birthday
Work/ leisure	Complete a poem I have been writing	Join a poetry group	Publish a book of poems

When completed, invite a few volunteers to share some items from their plans. End with a discussion by asking:

- » Is anyone surprised by what they have written?
- » Does having ambitious longer term goals provide more motivation?
- » If goals are totally unrealistic what effect might this have?
- » Do they think what they have written is achievable?
- » How does this make them feel?
- » What does this tell us about setting ourselves goals?

COMMENT

If anyone finds it difficult to set goals, suggest they fantasise about what they want to do.

HANDOUT: HAVING A GOAL

	Immediate	Reasonable	Wild
Personal			
Social			
Work/ leisure			

ROLES AND SKILLS

PURPOSE

To help group members identify the roles they have played and continue to play in life. It will also help people to think of themselves as individuals as well as value and put to use some of the skills they have accumulated over the year.

WHAT YOU'LL NEED

A whiteboard or flipchart, a marker, copies of the handout 'Roles and Skills' and pens.

WHAT TO DO

Explain that we all play a number of roles in everyday life. Brainstorm a list using a whiteboard or flipchart. Examples are:

» Son	» Car mechanic	» Handyman
» Daughter	» Diplomat	» Cleaner
» Father	» Teacher	» Boss
» Mother	» Friend	» Cook
» Gardener	» Secretary	» Mentor
» Nurse	» Lover	» Wife
» Soldier	» Carer	» Husband

Once a long list has been completed, give out the handout 'Roles and Skills' and instruct participants to fill in the roles they have played so far in life. When completed, ask everyone what skills they have acquired to fulfil these roles. Suggest they think about the skills they have most enjoyed using. Examples might be:

» Advising	» Organising	» Designing clothes
» Planning	» Researching	» Selling
» Growing plants	» Writing	» Making furniture
» Working with figures	» Bricklaying	» Teaching
» Listening	» Caring for people	» Computer technology

Split group members into pairs and ask them to work together helping each other to fill in five things they could now do with these skills in their current situation. Examples might be:

> » Work as a volunteer in a shop, library or animal sanctuary
>
> » Raise money for a charity
>
> » Organise family or community activities
>
> » Help at a youth club
>
> » Visit schools to talk about local history
>
> » Work for local or hospital radio
>
> » Become a volunteer hospital visitor
>
> » Organise a reading group

Bring people back together. Have a general discussion about the activity. Ask if they are surprised at the number of roles they have played and the skills they have acquired. How does that make them feel? Invite everyone, in turn, to share at least one of the five things they think they would like to do now with the skills they have acquired.

COMMENT

At the final stage of this activity, when participants consider how they can apply their skills, you may be able to raise possibilities such as taking up a new hobby or learning new skills to enable them to do something they have always wanted to do.

HANDOUT: ROLES AND SKILLS

Roles I have played in life are:

Skills I have acquired in these roles are:

Ways I can now use my skills and experiences are:

1.

2.

3.

4.

5.

A SNAPSHOT OF ME

PURPOSE

To raise awareness of how individuals see themselves at their current stage of life.

WHAT YOU'LL NEED

Sheets of paper, pens, pencils, markers and crayons.

WHAT TO DO

Give each person a sheet of paper divided into four sections with headings, as shown in the example below. Explain that doing this will give them a good view of how they see themselves now and how they would like things to progress. They will be able to refer back to it in six months' or a year's time to see how they have changed.

They can write simple words or sentences to express themselves in the spaces.

HOW I SEE MYSELF NOW	WHAT I'M PROUD ABOUT
Frightened Stuck in a maze Confused Uncertain about what to do	Retaining a sense of humour Keeping going My children
THINGS THAT MAKE ME FEEL GOOD	WHAT I WANT IN A YEAR'S TIME
Seeing my grandchildren Tea and a chat Playing the piano A good book	To be out of the maze To have completed my treatment To have sold my house and moved into a flat near my daughter

When the above has been completed, invite volunteers to show and talk briefly about their vision snapshot of themselves. Make it clear that anyone who doesn't want to share their vision of themselves does not have to do so.

COMMENT

You can call the snapshot 'A Picture of Me', 'A Shield', 'A Poster' or 'A Banner'. You can also give free rein for individuals to draw or use symbols such as matchstick figures or to use combinations of drawings and words to express themselves in the spaces.

WHERE I WANT TO BE

PURPOSE

To help individuals consider the direction in which they are going and what they need to do to get there.

WHAT YOU'LL NEED

Copies of the handout 'Where I Want to Be' and pens or pencils.

WHAT TO DO

Start by having an open discussion and asking participants questions such as:

» Is there anything you would like to do better?

» What else would you like to get out of life?

» Are you currently doing your very best?

» Is anything being wasted? Time, skills, knowledge, ability to learn, for example.

» What is stopping you? Could you do anything to overcome the problem?

» What qualities would you need to achieve what you want?

After the discussion, give out the handout 'Where I Want to Be' and ask participants to complete it. Suggest that before completing each section they sit back, close their eyes and imagine an answer to the question. They can either draw or write in the spaces provided.

When completed, bring everyone back together and invite anyone who feels comfortable doing so to share what they have written or drawn. Ask people how they feel now they have completed the exercise.

COMMENT

To maintain motivation and enthusiasm to move forward at any age it is necessary to be aware of personal qualities and to have goals – no matter how limiting the situation might be.

HANDOUT: WHERE I WANT TO BE

Where am I now?

Where do I want to be?

What is stopping me?

What qualities do I need to achieve my goals?

What realistic steps can I take?

LIVING YOUR IMAGINARY LIFE

PURPOSE

To create interest and motivation to fulfil an ambition.

WHAT YOU'LL NEED

Paper and pens or pencils.

WHAT TO DO

Explain that most people have had busy lives during which they have worked hard to gain qualifications, to earn a living, pay a mortgage or rent, raise and look after a family and then look after parents, and so on. During all that time, perhaps starting while at school, they may have wished for an imaginary life doing, or dabbling in art, writing novels, producing crafts, designing and making clothes, playing a musical instrument, singing in a choir, acting in a play, playing golf or bowls, doing yoga, learning to play chess, learning to dance and so on. Ask participants to call out a few examples of things they have had thoughts about over the years and would have liked to have had a go at.

Next, give out paper and pens and ask them to think back over their lives and write down five things they would have liked to have tried. When completed, split the group into pairs, who then discuss their imaginary life ambitions, and help each other decide which one of them they would like to have a go at and what they could do to take a first step towards achieving it in some way – perhaps join a group or class, buy a book on the subject, talk to someone who has experience in the subject and who might mentor them, for example. After a set time bring everyone back together and have each person, in turn, state what their imaginary life choice is and what they are going to do to bring it alive.

COMMENT

Individuals may sometimes chose subjects which they are not physically able to do, such as become a footballer, but they could still be involved with something to do with football.

I AM THE PERSON WHO…

PURPOSE

To retain confidence in abilities, preserve identity, maintain self-awareness and open up possibilities for the future.

WHAT YOU'LL NEED

Paper and pens or pencils.

WHAT TO DO

Give out paper and pens and ask participants to write a list of five things they do or have done in the past, each beginning with 'I am the person who…' For example:

1. *I am the person who writes poetry.*

2. *I am the person who does the garden.*

3. *I am the person who listens to people's problems.*

When completed, ask them to write another list, of five things they will do in the future. This time each sentence should begin with 'I am the person who will…' For example:

1. *I am the person who will go for a walk in the garden this afternoon.*

2. *I am the person who will bake a cake for my grand-daughter's birthday next week.*

3. *I am the person who will put together my family history.*

When this list is finished, invite participants to share and discuss at least one item from each of their lists. Encourage other group members to ask questions and give encouragement about the information shared.

COMMENT

You can increase or decrease the number of things you ask people to write on their lists according to how challenging you want to make the activity.

DIFFICULT TOPICS

ACTIVITIES TO HELP DISCUSS
TOPICS WHICH CAN BE
DIFFICULT TO TALK ABOUT

NEGATIVE AND POSITIVE THOUGHTS AND FEELINGS

PURPOSE

To aid the expression of negative and positive thoughts and feelings.

WHAT YOU'LL NEED

A flipchart or whiteboard and marker. Pens and paper if doing it as a writing exercise.

WHAT TO DO

Explain that we all experience negative and unpleasant feelings from time to time. Often they may make us feel guilty or inadequate. These may be feelings around changes in health, circumstances or experiences past, present or future. Knowing that these feelings are normal doesn't make them go away. We need to deal with them in a constructive way.

Write the word 'worry' on a flipchart or whiteboard. Ask everyone to consider what the words mean to them in the context of their current situation. Give an example: 'I'm worried about my brother. He isn't in the best of health. I think I should be doing more to help him but he lives over 200 miles away and I don't drive.'

Now give each person, in turn, an opportunity to state something that worries them. They can expand on it if they wish and other group members can be invited to comment on how they deal with similar feelings. In a large group you might need to limit the amount of time spent discussing each statement.

Other words you can use for a second or third round are:

> » Regret

> » Guilt

> » Embarrassment

> » Irritation

> » Shame

> » Anger

> » Hate

> » Disgust

Next, to avoid leaving any group members with negative feelings, repeat the same exercise with words that inspire positive thoughts. Here are a few:

- » Love
- » Tranquillity
- » Loyalty
- » Friendship
- » Enthusiasm
- » Enjoyment
- » Peace
- » Excitement

COMMENT

Of course, you can use different words on different occasions so that over a period of time you cover many different thoughts and feelings experienced by participants. This can also be done as a writing exercise. Give participants an allotted time to write down their thoughts about what the word means to them. After the set period, invite individuals to read out and discuss what they have written.

OVERCOMING THE STIGMA OF DAILY LIVING AIDS

PURPOSE

To explore personal perceptions and feelings about using daily living devices.

WHAT YOU'LL NEED

Compile a list of and obtain pictures and stories, where possible, of people of all ages from different walks of life who use daily living aids and have been very successful. This might include Olympic sports champions, ex-armed forces or people who have overcome disability to raise money for charity. Collect as many examples as possible from papers, magazines and books. Also use Google to obtain examples. You will also need a flipchart or whiteboard and markers, paper and pens.

WHAT TO DO

Explain that age brings with it the need to use devices such as wheelchairs, hearing and walking aids, grab rails, GPS trackers and personal hygiene aids. People often make judgements about people using these devices. These prejudices can influence personal attitudes towards making use of them and how individuals feel about themselves.

Start a discussion about how family, friends and people in the community view people who use aids. Ask:

» What conclusions might friends and other people in the community draw about someone using aids? Do they see the aid or the person? (Note on a whiteboard both negative and positive comments.)

» What are your feelings about using the devices? (Again, note negative and positive comments.)

» What benefits do you get from using the aids? (Write on the board.)

Pass around the pictures and stories about people who use aids and have become very successful. Or have them displayed on a table and ask people to circulate and look at them. Then ask:

» What qualities and abilities do you see in these people that are more important than the devices? What enables you to see them as people? (Write some on the board.)

Next, give out some paper and pens and ask participants to write down five qualities and abilities they have – things people can see in them as individuals, rather than focusing on the aids. When completed, invite group members to share their qualities.

COMMENT

You can do this activity without the pictures and stories about successful people but you will need to ensure you emphasise that the devices enable people of all ages to lead very successful and fulfilling lives.

ACKNOWLEDGING FEELINGS

PURPOSE

To help people identify, acknowledge and express uncomfortable feelings and share ideas on ways of dealing with them.

WHAT YOU'LL NEED

Copies of the handout 'Acknowledging Feelings' and pens.

WHAT TO DO

Explain that we are often unaware of how we are feeling at any given time. Say that it is easy to become slightly detached from our emotions, other people and ourselves. This can occur because:

» As a child we may have put our own feelings aside to meet the demands of a needy parent.

» We like to gain approval from other people so focus mainly on how others are feeling.

» We switch off our own feelings because we have been hurt emotionally and see feelings as painful and dangerous.

» We were brought up in a family where feelings were kept hidden.

» We keep busy so we don't have to face our own feelings.

» We focus on the intellectual side of life and do not talk about feelings.

Say that the exercise you are about to do is aimed at helping people identify, express and deal with their emotions. Give out the handout 'Acknowledging Feelings', explain how to fill it in and ask individuals to complete it.

When completed, invite participants, in turn, to share some of their feelings, body sensations and how they have dealt with this. Encourage everyone to share ideas about how they cope with their emotions.

End the activity by pointing out that by getting to know our emotions better we can see that they are there for a reason. No matter how distressing they might be, they are a part of being human. When we acknowledge and find language to express them we can find ways to live with them.

COMMENT

The 'Dealing with Feelings' section of the handout can be deleted. You can then cover this by having a general discussion, with everyone sharing some of their feelings and how they handle them.

HANDOUT: ACKNOWLEDGING FEELINGS

Tick or circle five feelings you have experienced during the past week. Blank spaces are provided for feelings not listed.

jealous	angry	loved	worried
frightened	unloved	satisfied	bored
confused	threatened	sad	abandoned
needy	ashamed	anxious	embarrassed
lost	trapped	hurt	misunderstood
powerless	rejected	lonely	frustrated
guilty	irritated	resentful	outraged
happy	useless	proud	bitter
agitated	vulnerable	overwhelmed	miserable
numb	fulfilled	envious	joyful

BODY SENSATIONS

Tick or circle any of the body sensations which accompanied the feelings experienced. Blank spaces are provided for sensations not listed.

tearful	cold	migraine	shaky
sweaty	frail	dizzy	backache
tired	difficulty breathing	nauseous	clenched fists
headache	explosive	heart racing	apathetic
hungry	tight	neck aches	sweaty palms
wobbly	feverish	buzzing	floppy

DEALING WITH FEELINGS

Complete the following:

Feelings experienced	How this affected me (body sensations)	How I deal with these feelings
1.		
2.		
3.		
4.		
5.		

FEELING SAFE

PURPOSE

To articulate concerns relating to feeling safe when out and about and explore some solutions.

WHAT YOU'LL NEED

Make up some fictional newspaper headings or cut some from a local paper and display them to set the tone. For example: 'Man trips on uneven pavement', 'Youth steals handbag', 'Is it safe on the streets at night?', 'Woman gets lost on way home', 'Man boards wrong bus'. Make these appropriate to fears that people in the group might have in their particular situations. You will also need a whiteboard or flipchart and a marker.

WHAT TO DO

Briefly introduce the topic and then invite group members to call out things which worry them when they are out and about. Make a list of fears on a board or flipchart. When completed, break participants into two or three subgroups. Split the fears up between the subgroups. They then discuss the fears and what actions might be taken to deal with the situations. For example, if a person fears losing their way when returning home, they might carry a card with their name and address and/or a street map showing the way with landmarks marked on it. After a set time, bring the group back together and have each subgroup present their set of fears/problems and possible solutions.

End by inviting group members who originally voiced the fears if they would feel able to use any of the proposed solutions to enable them to feel safer when out and about.

COMMENT

Some of the proposed solutions may be out of the control of group members, for example, fixing uneven pavements and poor streetlighting or increasing police visibility. In these instances ask the group if there is any way they could exert influence, such as writing to the council and/or a local paper as a group, or working with the residential home management, a local neighbourhood group or the police. This avoids participants feeling helpless and unable to influence the situation. It also adds to their feelings of self-worth.

You can also focus this activity specifically on group members feeling safe in their home, or in their residential or nursing home.

CLARIFYING MY END-OF-LIFE WISHES

PURPOSE

To provide an opportunity for thought and discussion on end-of-life care and preferences and ways to communicate these wishes to loved ones and others involved in their care.

WHAT YOU'LL NEED

Copies of the handout 'Clarifying My End-of-Life Wishes' and pens.

WHAT TO DO

Explain that throughout life we celebrate or talk about events such as births, getting married, retirement, and so on, and safe sex and drugs, but rarely discuss how we want to be cared for if we become seriously ill or what our wishes are as we approach the end of life. That is, until we are in crisis and then it adds to the difficulty and becomes overwhelming. Ask participants:

» Have they made a will or discussed their preferences for future care with anyone? If not, why not?

» When do they think is the best time to do this: before or after illness or a crisis occurs?

Split the participants into small groups and give each person a copy of the handout 'Clarifying My End-of-Life Wishes'. Instruct each of the subgroups to discuss what their wishes are regarding the topics listed and make notes on the sheet for their own use. (The topics are only intended to get them thinking. Participants may wish to add other issues.)

After a set time, bring everyone back together. Ask participants how they feel after their discussion and invite them to share some of their ideas about how they can go about communicating their wishes to their family and others as necessary.

COMMENT

Make it clear that participants should seek professional advice about making wills, appointing power of attorney or other legal documents. The activity is to help individuals clarify for themselves what they want before formalising it. Over time, individuals may change their minds about what they want. These changes will also need to be communicated to loved ones and others involved in their care.

HANDOUT: CLARIFYING MY END-OF-LIFE WISHES

MY WISHES
People I need to discuss my wishes with are:
Care if I become ill: Be cared for at home or in a hospice? Be resuscitated or not? Organ donation? Emotional and spiritual support I would like:
Legal: Will completed and up to date? Power of attorney for finance and/or healthcare appointed? Who?

MY WISHES

Funeral:
Cremation or burial?

What type of service? (Include details about location, music, flowers, memorials, etc.)

Other information:

Ways I can best communicate my wishes to my family and others are:

HIDDEN FEELINGS

PURPOSE

To help people identify, acknowledge and express hidden feelings and share ideas for expressing them.

WHAT YOU'LL NEED

A whiteboard or flipchart, marker, pens and paper.

WHAT TO DO

Hidden feelings are those feelings that we keep to ourselves, often for fear of offending family members, friends or acquaintances with whom we are in regular contact. The fact is that – despite their initial surprise – when we own and communicate our true feelings, values and opinions, people usually feel safer and more secure with us. The relationship becomes more honest. Also, the truth often surprises us ourselves.

Ask participants:

» Have there been occasions when you have kept your feelings or opinions to yourself rather than acknowledge or voice them? (Ask for examples.)

» Are there times when not voicing them is the right action? (Ask for examples.)

» When is voicing them the correct action?

After discussion, write the following on the board or a flipchart:

'I go along with _____ but actually I feel _____.'

('I go along with *my partner expecting me to do all the cleaning* but actually I feel *resentful and that he/she is taking advantage. He/she should do an equal amount.*')

Now give out paper and pens and ask participants to write down, using the words above, five separate occasions when they have gone along with something or someone else's vision of what they feel when, actually, they feel quite differently.

When completed, split the participants into subgroups of two or three people. These subgroups now share what they have written, and discuss whether or not they should voice their real feelings and how they might go about doing that.

End the activity by bringing everyone back together and inviting each subgroup to give at least one example of a hidden feeling and what they have decided is the appropriate action to help the person voice their real feelings. Allow other group members to add their comments.

COMMENT

These hidden feelings can create tensions, poison relationships and make life unpleasant. Being honest and facing our true feelings empowers us.

THROW YOUR WORRIES AWAY

PURPOSE

To enable participants to share worries and obtain different responses to the concern.

WHAT YOU'LL NEED

Paper, pens and an empty box or basket.

WHAT TO DO

State that participants will now have an opportunity to throw away their worries or concerns. Invite each person to think and write down a question, worry, problem or concern. This might be about a topic being addressed in the group, a task to be undertaken such as a craft or art project, changes being made to something or life in general. After they have written down their particular worry, ask them to crinkle up their paper and throw it into a basket or box which has been placed in the centre of the room.

When all the crumpled pieces of paper are in the box, ask one group member to pick one out and toss it to anyone in the room. This person opens the paper and reads the worry out loud. Participants then discuss possible options or solutions to the problem. Make it clear that whoever wrote about the worry does not have to disclose their identity unless they wish to do so. Repeat the procedure until all the worries have been addressed.

COMMENT

You can use this activity at the beginning of a session, at any time during it or at the end. It usually brings out worries that participants find difficult or are normally reluctant to bring up or speak about.

ASKING FOR HELP

PURPOSE

To help individuals acknowledge areas in which they need help and to ask for it

WHAT YOU'LL NEED

A whiteboard or a flipchart and a marker. Copies of the handout 'Asking for Help' and pens or pencils.

WHAT TO DO

Explain that asking for help can be really hard and then discuss what difficulties group members have around asking for help. Write these on the whiteboard or flipchart under the heading 'Barriers'. This may include the following fears:

» *Being turned down.* (Remind participants that most people enjoy helping. It makes them feel good. The worst that can happen is that the person says 'no'. But it might just be that one particular thing they feel unable to do, or uncomfortable about. They may well be very willing to do something else to assist.)

» *Being a burden.* (Do these boil down to fears about the future, feeling you are not worth the effort of others? It also makes the assumption that the person helping thinks of it as a burden. They might just think of it as part of a caring friendship or loving relationship and find it meaningful.)

» *Admitting they are having difficulty coping.* (Suggest they try thinking about the problem as if it is an object. Imagine you and someone else teaming up against 'it'. This (problem) needs to get sorted before 'it' makes their life even more difficult.)

» *Owing a favour or feeling indebted.* (They could try switching feelings of indebtedness to one of appreciation for the help. 'Thank you! Your help has really made life so much easier.' If someone instils a feeling of obligation or manipulation, look for a different helper.)

» *Appearing weak or inadequate.* (Suggest they remind themselves that we all need help and support at times. Being able to ask for help when needed is a sign of strength, not weakness. Having someone to ask means you are connected and supported. They could also try to reframe their problem as consulting with someone who they trust to do a good job.)

Now ask about what makes it easier to ask for help, and write these on the board. This might include:

» Knowing the type of help you need

» Talking through the situation with someone

» Accepting that giving and taking is part of life

» Realising that there are situations in which one can help oneself and others when one needs help from others

» Being able to open up and trust someone

After the discussion, give out the handout 'Asking For Help' and ask participants to complete it in the order in which the sections are numbered. Things they need help with might include: shopping, particular errands, changing a light bulb, walking the dog, help getting dressed/undressed, trimming the hedge or having someone to chat to.

When thinking about people who might help, participants should consider friends, relatives and professionals such as social workers or care workers. When picking the person most suited to a task, participants should bear in bear in mind the chosen person's strengths, the time they have available and their own comfort with the person, depending on the intimacy of the task.

When completed, ask participants who feel comfortable doing so to share the task they have chosen to ask for help with. How do they feel about doing it? Discuss any fears. Point out that once this first request for help has been actioned they can then choose a second task and ask for help with that.

COMMENT

Asking for help is difficult for most people. We frequently blame others for not seeing we need it and offering it, and procrastinate or refuse to accept help until our problem has developed into an emergency.

HANDOUT: ASKING FOR HELP

Things I need help with are:

People who might help are:

The people most suited to these tasks are: (Choose from the list of people who might help.)

Pick one thing off the list you need assistance with and write down what you will say to potential helpers. Be direct. (Instead of saying, 'If only I could get someone to put the rubbish bins out for collection', ask directly: 'Would you put the rubbish bins out for collection for me, please? I'm not yet strong enough to manage them.')

MAKING DECISIONS

PURPOSE

To discuss the effects of making or not making decisions and explore the difficulties.

WHAT YOU'LL NEED

Whiteboard or flipchart and a marker.

WHAT TO DO

Introduce the activity by asking participants to quickly share a decision they have made today. This might be something like what to have for breakfast or to what to wear.

Now write two columns on a board or flipchart, heading one 'Easy Decisions' and the other 'Difficult Decisions'. Invite participants to call out the type of decisions – both easy and difficult – they are now facing or might be faced with in the future. These could be anything from making a will to having an operation or a birthday party – the details should not be discussed.

When completed, ask why some decisions are easy and others are difficult. Then guide the discussion so that it covers the types of things that should be considered before making a decision. These should include:

» Will anyone else influence these decisions?

» Will the outcome affect anyone else?

» Are there any consequences of the outcome for the decision-maker?

» What changes might occur as a result?

» What would be the outcome of not making any decision?

» Should things be discussed with anyone or advice be sought with anyone before taking action?

End the activity by asking individuals, in turn, to state a decision they made in the past with which they are pleased. This might be anything from getting married (or divorced) to having a holiday or changing their job.

COMMENT

Decisions can become very difficult as people become older. There is the temptation to put things off or ignore them, hoping that they will go away.

A PROBLEM SHARED

PURPOSE

To dispel natural fears about ageing and to promote individual wellbeing.

WHAT YOU'LL NEED

A whiteboard or flipchart and a marker.

WHAT TO DO

Explain that as individuals age it is natural to have fears about ageing and the common problems this brings. This can include difficulty hearing, some visual impairment, joint pains, being unable to sleep and being unable to do some things.

Invite participants to share details of their difficulties and any solutions they have found which help. Solutions might include relaxing with soft music before going to sleep, taking a short stroll before breakfast to help with arthritis, turning the radio or TV off when talking to someone to help with hearing, and using an alarm or a written note to remember to do something.

You can write the problems discussed on a whiteboard or flipchart, together with some of the solutions offered. End the activity by asking if anyone is going to try some of the ideas.

COMMENT

You will be surprised that even the quietest members of the group will be drawn into making a contribution. Do make it clear that for medical advice individuals should speak to a medical practitioner. You will find that open discussion will promote individual insight and tolerance of their problems.

CREATIVITY

ACTIVITIES TO MAINTAIN
CREATIVE ABILITIES

STORY IN A BAG

PURPOSE

To stimulate creativity, use of the imagination and conversation through the use of story telling.

WHAT YOU'LL NEED

Four to six objects in a bag, one bag for each subgroup. Objects might include a book, a glove, a paper-knife, a lipstick, a scarf, a paperweight, a pen, a diary or a shoe. The more diverse the better.

WHAT TO DO

Divide the participants into small subgroups of three or four people. Give each subgroup a bag. Allow participants ten or fifteen minutes to create a story that incorporates all the items. They can be as inventive as they please and make it a romance, murder, fantasy, comedy or any other style of story.

When the stories have been completed, invite each subgroup in turn to present their story to everyone. Explain that different group members can tell different parts of the story or they can act it out making it as dramatic and entertaining as possible. Give them a moment or two to prepare and then begin the presentations.

COMMENT

A really excellent activity that is good fun, makes everyone smile, breaks down barriers and gets everyone talking. For less able groups you might need to allow more time.

FORTUNATELY/UNFORTUNATELY

PURPOSE

To stimulate imagination, practise flexible thinking and have fun.

WHAT YOU'LL NEED

No materials needed but you will need to think of a beginning sentence for the story.

WHAT TO DO

Start a story beginning with the word *fortunately*. The person sitting next to you then continues the story with a sentence beginning with the word *unfortunately*. The person next to them starts the next sentence starting with the word *fortunately*. The story is built sentence by sentence alternating the words *fortunately* and *unfortunately* as each person takes a turn. Individuals add only one sentence. It might go something like:

> You: *Fortunately, I won the lottery and bought a house on a cliff at the seaside.*

> Next person: *Unfortunately, the cliff and house fell into the sea in the night.*

> Next person: *Fortunately, I was saved by a man in a passing boat.*

> Next person: *Unfortunately, he was an escaped convict from the prison further along the coast who took me as a hostage.*

> Next person: *Fortunately, the police were in hot pursuit.*

> Next person: *Unfortunately, we crashed into the town pier.*

> Next person: *Fortunately, I could swim.*

> Next person: *Unfortunately, we were attacked by a shark.*

The story continues in this fashion until everyone has added to the story. If it is a small group you can pass the story round the group two or three times.

COMMENT

Keeping the contributions to one sentence ensures that the story keeps building. Also, the sudden twists add to the entertainment. A variation would be to give each person a sheet of paper with a beginning sentence and a list of statements to be filled in down the sheet. For example:

Fortunately: *I met someone and fell in love while on holiday in Russia.*

Unfortunately:

Fortunately:

Unfortunately:

And so on down the sheet.

Participants then fill in the next sentence and pass the sheet on to the person on their left who fills in the following blank sentence. This continues until everyone has completed at least one sentence on each sheet. The stories are then read out.

PROVERBS

PURPOSE

To stimulate creative thinking and the ability to use analogy.

WHAT YOU'LL NEED

A whiteboard or a flipchart and a marker, and a list of common proverbs such as:

Barking dogs seldom bite

It's never too late to learn

Every cloud has a silver lining

Two heads are better than one

One man's meat is another man's poison

Absence makes the heart grow fonder

Don't count your chickens before they're hatched

A friend in need is a friend indeed

WHAT TO DO

Invite participants to call out well-known proverbs. Write these on a whiteboard or flipchart. Choose one or two and discuss what they mean. For example:

Proverb: *Those who live in glass houses should not throw stones.*

Meaning: *We should not blame other people for faults we ourselves possess. Glass houses are easily damaged. So, if you throw stones at a neighbour's glass house they will throw stones back and damage your home.*

Ask if anyone can think of examples of the proverb meaning or can make up an imaginary story that bears out the meaning. Once everyone is clear about how to make an analogy, split participants into subgroups of three or four people. Give each subgroup a proverb and instruct them to make up a story to illustrate it. They can base it on a real-life event if they wish.

When the subgroups have completed their stories, invite each one, in turn, to tell their story. Other group members then guess what the proverb might be.

COMMENT

Instead of asking the subgroups to just make up and relate a story illustrating the proverb, instruct them to plan and act out a short improvised drama.

TRUE OR FALSE

PURPOSE

To stimulate imagination, creativity and quick thinking.

WHAT YOU'LL NEED

Ask each participant to bring along a personal object such as a handbag, an ornament, a rock, a piece of jewellery, a drawing, a book, a picture, a scarf or a medal.

WHAT TO DO

There may or may not be a true story which has happened involving the object. Invite group members, in turn, to show their object and relate a story about it. The story can be as mundane or as fantastic as the person likes to make it. Allow a moment or two for thought and then invite a volunteer to begin. For example, if the object was a necktie the person might say something like:

> 'This is tie which was given to me in the summer of 1963 by Marlene Dietrich when she was in London. At the time I worked in a menswear department store. She came into the store and bought two dozen ties. She said she wanted them to give as presents to anyone who did something for her such as opening a door or carrying parcels. When she was leaving the store it was raining. I escorted her to her car, covering her with an umbrella. As a thank-you she gave me one of the ties she had just bought. This is that tie.'

Other group members now vote by raising a hand on whether they think the story is true or false.

COMMENT

You can extend this activity by, before voting, inviting the other group members to ask the story teller questions after each story has been related. A variation would be to supply the objects and ask each person to select one and make up a story about it. After stories are related, the other members can then vote on which they think was the most imaginative and give the winner a simple prize.

Group members can also be split into small subgroups to make up a story and present it. The participants then vote for which story is best. They are, of course, not allowed to vote for their own story.

SEEING THE FUNNY SIDE OF LIFE

PURPOSE

To add humour, stimulate creative thinking and bring out the funny side of life.

WHAT YOU'LL NEED

Sheets of paper, glue, scissors, a range of magazines and newspapers, pens or pencils.

WHAT TO DO

Lay out a range of magazines and newspapers and invite participants to browse through them and cut out a couple of pictures of celebrities or politicians, footballers, people in the news, animals, cartoon characters, and so on. It may even be one picture showing a few people. Using a glue stick, participants then stick their chosen figures on a sheet of paper. They then draw a speech bubble from each person's mouth and write funny speech comments in them. When everyone is ready, invite each person, in turn, to show and explain their chosen pictures.

COMMENT

If using scissors presents a problem or danger to participants, cut the figures out beforehand and lay the pictures out on a table for them to choose from. Having them cut their own figures out usually works best, however, as there is often an article in the magazine or paper about the famous person which gives a context on which to base the humorous speech comments.

MAKE UP A STORY

PURPOSE

To stimulate creativity by making connections between different things.

WHAT YOU'LL NEED

Copies of the handout 'Make Up a Story'.

WHAT TO DO

Give participants copies of the handout 'Make Up a Story' and instruct them to randomly pick one element from each of the columns so they have 'two characters', 'an emotion' and 'an object'.

Each person then makes up a story, using the elements chosen. For example, they might randomly choose 'Schoolboy', 'Friend', 'Jealousy' and 'A mobile phone'. The story might go something like:

Jason overhears a mate, Peter, phoning a girl he (Jason) is in love with and asking her out to see a film. Jealous, Jason later phones Peter and tells him his Dad has had an accident and he needs to get to the hospital. While Peter is at the hospital, Jason meets up with the girl and says he will go to see the film with her. When they come out of the cinema, Peter is waiting for them and tells Jason that he is a creep. The girl then says that she really liked Jason but now thinks he is a nasty piece of work and Peter and she are only friends. She tells him to get lost and walks off with Peter.

It doesn't have to be a great story. It is a fun activity to stimulate the imagination. After a few minutes for thought, invite participants, in turn, to relate their stories.

COMMENT

You can split participants into pairs or groups of three and get the groups to choose the elements and make up the stories. And, of course, you can create your own list of elements from which participants can choose. This can also be used as a writing activity.

HANDOUT: MAKE UP A STORY

1st character	2nd character	An emotion	An object
Doctor	Grandad	Anger	A mobile phone
Gardener	Stepmother	Denial	A gun
Musician	Bridesmaid	Love	A bouquet
Footballer	Friend	Jealousy	A diamond
Burglar	Lover	Resentment	A walking stick
Pop star	Waitress	Impatience	A knife
Soldier	Grand-daughter	Revenge	A car
Schoolboy	Police officer	Envy	A computer
Plumber	Girlfriend	Guilt	A bicycle
Chef	A baby	Pride	A key
Boxer	Stepson	Hatred	A football
Secret agent	Drug addict	Fear	A boat

MATCHING INTERESTS AND SKILLS

PURPOSE

To spark creativity when thinking of new things to do.

WHAT YOU'LL NEED

Sheets of paper and pens or pencils.

WHAT TO DO

Instruct participants to write a numbered list of ten things they enjoy doing. This might be activities such as swimming, listening to music, reading thrillers, knitting or jigsaw puzzles. Next, ask them to write down another numbered list of ten skills they possess. For example, cooking, talking to children, organising, drawing, telling jokes or singing.

Next, call out two numbers between one and ten. Each person now links the two numbers on their lists and comes up with something new they could do. For example, the activity and skills of reading thrillers and organising might combine to inspire the person to organise a thriller-reading group to meet once a month. Swimming and drawing might combine to inspire the person to produce sketches at the local beach or river. Continue in this manner until everyone has come up with at least five new things they could do.

End the activity by having each person, in turn, state something new they intend having a go at.

COMMENT

This is a fun way to stimulate creative ideas. The activity also works well when participants are split into pairs to help each other with ideas.

SOLVE THAT PROBLEM

PURPOSE

To practise using creative thinking to come up with solutions to problems and have fun.

WHAT YOU'LL NEED

Pens and paper so that people can write their ideas down, and a whiteboard or flipchart and marker.

WHAT TO DO

Write two or three problems on the whiteboard or flipchart for participants to solve. For example:

> » Someone stealing plants from gardens

> » Two people always arguing

Also provide five random words, such as Science, Oil, Sea, Love and Rash.

Split the participants into small groups of three or four people and instruct them to choose one of the problems and use one of the words to come up with a solution to it. They can also think up other solutions using the other words – one word for each solution. For example:

Problem: Noise from a local club late at night as revellers walk home through the streets.

Random words: Phantom, Fish, Italy, Bus, Magic.

Possible solutions:

1. *Get the local bus service to provide a **bus** to take people home (so they don't walk through the surrounding streets).*

2. *Create a story about a **phantom** big cat that haunts the area late at night and get it published in the local paper to deter people from walking through the area.*

After a set time, have the subgroups present their solutions to everyone. End by discussing how it felt doing the activity. Ask if it gave them any ideas about expanding their thinking concerning solving everyday problems.

COMMENT

The more random words you provide for groups to use, the easier it is to come up with possible solutions.

STORY ENDINGS

PURPOSE

To use imagination, work together, exercise creative thinking and have fun.

WHAT YOU'LL NEED

Have the beginning of a story in mind. Have a TV and recorder available if using the TV option.

WHAT TO DO

Split the group into subgroups of three or four people. Make up a story beginning or tell a story beginning taken from a magazine, newspaper, book or a play. The members of each subgroup, working together, then work out what happens in the rest of the story, bringing it to a satisfactory conclusion. When completed, each subgroup relates their story to the whole group.

COMMENT

You'll be surprised at the variety of stories which emanate from the same beginning. Alternatively, invite participants to watch the beginning of a soap opera or TV programme and then get them to complete the episode. If you limit the characters in the stories to the same number of people as in the subgroups you can get them to perform one or two or all of the scenes they have created.

SCENES FROM LIFE

PURPOSE

To stimulate creativity, use imagination and memory.

WHAT YOU'LL NEED

A number of figures of animals, birds, people or objects cut from magazines. Art materials, including glue.

WHAT TO DO

Lay the figures out on a table and ask participants to choose one. They then glue this at the centre of a sheet of paper and then, by drawing, painting or using coloured pencils, create a scene around the figure. If a sheep, this may be on a mountainside; if a bird it could be in a town garden; or, if a person, they may be walking down a street or be at a horseracing event. Ask them to outline what is suggested to them by the figure.

End by inviting everyone to show and talk about their picture.

COMMENT

To stimulate memories of the past you could choose objects and figures from a particular era. For example: an old tractor, truck or motorcycle, a boy on a bike from the 1960s or 1970s, a woman dressed 1950s fashion, a soldier from the Second World War, or an old radio or gramophone.

OUR MAGAZINE

PURPOSE

To work together creatively and have fun.

WHAT YOU'LL NEED

Large sheets of paper and felt pens so that the subgroups can write down their ideas.

WHAT TO DO

Form subgroups of four or five people. Advise participants that they are going to be given a task to complete. Tell them that your organisation has decided that you are going to start producing a monthly magazine for the people the organisation supports and their relatives. The task for each group is to decide what the magazine will contain and who might write in it. Who might they approach to produce each item? This could include articles, information, interviews, cartoons, puzzles, pictures, news, poetry. The items chosen should be realistic. Set a limited time, say 20 or 30 minutes, for them to decide the contents.

When the time is up, a member from each subgroup gives a presentation of what they have decided and the reason why each item will be included. After the presentations ask participants:

> » Was it difficult to come to a consensus?

> » How did they resolve differences of opinion?

> » Could good ideas from different groups be incorporated together to improve each group's presentation?

> » What does this tell us about sharing problems and working together to resolve them?

COMMENT

The task does not have to be designing a magazine. It could be anything else relevant to the group members, such as planning a birthday party, an outing, a gardening project, a celebration, an activity programme for an open day, putting on a musical evening or a menu for a surprise meal. If the task is one which can be realised it provides real incentive and enthusiasm.

COMMUNICATION

ACTIVITIES TO SUPPORT AND IMPROVE COMMUNICATION SKILLS

WHAT QUALITY OF LIFE MEANS FOR ME

PURPOSE

To enable individuals to express what is important to them.

WHAT YOU'LL NEED

A whiteboard or flipchart, pens and paper.

WHAT TO DO

Explain that quality of life includes the right for everyone to live life in the way that they wish without harming other people. To do this we need to look forward to the future and communicate to our families and friends what we want and how we wish to live.

1. Ask group members to discuss and say what is important to maintain a good quality of life. The suggestions can be written on a whiteboard or flipchart. This might include being able to:

   » Maintain dignity

   » Be respected

   » Practise their faith

   » Have companionship

   » Stay independent

   » Make own choices

   » Be secure

   » Take part in family life

2. Now hand out paper and pens and instruct participants to think for a moment and list three things which they want in future as part of their life. They can start with the words:

   Three things I want in the future are:

   (a)

   (b)

   (c)

3. When completed, invite each group member, in turn, to share at least one of their wishes. As they share them, ask if this is something they can achieve for themselves or if they will need assistance. Discuss. Encourage other group members to suggest ways in which they might ask for assistance to help carry out their wishes.

COMMENT

Many of the things people want in order to maintain their quality of life are fairly simple and straightforward to put in place, and it can make such a difference to their lives.

STARTING CONVERSATIONS

PURPOSE

To encourage individuals to develop new relationships and gain confidence opening conversations.

WHAT YOU'LL NEED

A whiteboard or flipchart and markers.

WHAT TO DO

Begin by facilitating a discussion about the type of situations in which individuals find it difficult to initiate conversations. Note these on a whiteboard or flipchart so everyone can see them. They will come up with statements such as:

» Discussing something that has happened in the news

» Asking a question about the other person

» Giving a compliment

» Commenting on what is going to happen during the day

» Talking about something that has happened to them

» Talking about something new they are going to do

» Asking someone how they are

» Discussing something they have just done

When you have listed a fair number of situations, divide the group into pairs or small subgroups. Give two or three listed situations to each subgroup. Instruct them to write down the subjects and discuss suggestions for opening sentences that would help start a conversation or keep it going in those circumstances. They can use flipchart sheets to do this. Suggestions might include:

How are you feeling today?

My name is...

Today I'm going to...

I'm starting to find it difficult to...

Wasn't the flooding shown on TV last night terrible?

I feel a bit down today. My son has...

I didn't sleep well. I would like you to...

That's really interesting. Can you tell me...?

When a set time has passed, get each subgroup, in turn, to show their flipchart sheets and share both their situations and the conversation solutions they have discussed. The sheets can be displayed on the walls.

Next, ask people to select another partner. Then instruct them to practise starting up a conversation using a combination of any of the suggestions for subjects to talk about and the opening sentences. After a few minutes, stop the proceedings and ask them to move on to a new partner. They then use a different subject and opening sentence. Move people on to new partners three of four times.

Finally, assemble everyone in a circle and ask them how the conversations went. How did they feel? How could the conversations be improved?

COMMENT

There are many reasons why older people may find it difficult to open conversations. These may include:

- » Being withdrawn and isolated
- » Feeling they have little or nothing to contribute
- » Disliking asking for help
- » Loss of confidence
- » Being unable to hear properly
- » Feeling angry
- » Feeling stigmatised

Often individuals will need assistance overcoming these obstacles. You may need to discuss and identify with each person what their particular difficulties are and address them.

PICTURE CHARADES

PURPOSE

To communicate non-verbally, work with others to solve problems and have fun.

WHAT YOU'LL NEED

A whiteboard or flipchart and a marker, or drawing paper and felt tip pens. It is also helpful to have a list of animals or creatures in mind for individuals who have difficulty thinking on the spot. Examples might be: octopus, zebra, camel, lion, ant, elephant, alligator, kangaroo, butterfly, rabbit, moose, whale, cat, dog.

WHAT TO DO

Invite a group member to draw on the board the picture outline of an animal or creature. Other participants then try to guess what it is. The artist must not give any hints or clues to what they are drawing except to answer 'yes' or 'no' when the group tries to guess. Repeat this process with each member of the group until everyone has had a turn.

COMMENT

Other categories you could use are vegetables, flowers or famous landmarks, such as the Eiffel Tower. If you use more difficult categories, such as landmarks or types of tree, it is useful to have pictures available for the artist to see as they draw. As an alternative, space participants a little distance apart and give each person a sheet of drawing paper, a felt tip pen and a slip of paper with a subject written on it for them to draw. When all the drawings are complete, each person, in turn, shows their drawing and the other group members guess what it is.

TALKING STICK

PURPOSE

To enhance group communication, create a format for uninterrupted disclosure and emphasise listening as a necessary part of communication.

WHAT YOU'LL NEED

A stick and some topics on which it is important that people express their opinions. Although you can use any sort of stick – even a ruler – it is best if it looks special. Colour and decorate it with feathers or ribbons. Topics can be around local issues, things in the news, TV programmes, issues in the day centre or home or topics participants want to discuss.

WHAT TO DO

Explain that the idea of a talking stick is taken from the custom of Native Americans. Elders use it when meeting to discuss important tribal issues. The stick is passed around the circle, allowing each person to speak and be heard without being interrupted. When holding the stick you can speak and put your point, observations or feelings across. When not holding the stick you listen and concentrate on understanding what is being said. There is no obligation to speak when holding the stick. (Make sure everyone understands this.) If you don't have anything to say, hold it briefly to see if anything comes to mind and, if not, pass it on. If time permits, pass the stick round the circle twice and then place it in the centre. Encourage anyone who has more to say to take the stick and speak and then return it to the centre. When people are holding the stick, allow periods for silence and reflection rather than rushing on to the next person.

Once everyone understands how the system works, introduce the topic to be discussed and start the process.

COMMENT

You can just pass the stick and ask each person to talk about anything that comes to mind, is causing them concern or they want to share. This can initiate some interesting sessions. You can also use the stick as a means of getting people to reflect on the session: 'Let's reflect on what we have done today' or 'What are you going to do differently as a result of what you have learned today?'

In groups with good cohesion and when trust has been established, people will usually share thoughtful and personal information. Being able to speak without being interrupted allows them to voice their innermost feelings and thoughts. People who tend to monopolise discussions may find it difficult remaining silent. You may need to discuss this at the end of the activity. Also, ask if anyone felt uncomfortable, and why.

IMPROVING LISTENING SKILLS

PURPOSE

To work on listening skills as an aid to maintaining communication and social interactions.

WHAT YOU'LL NEED

A whiteboard or flipchart, a marker, paper and pens for the observers and some appropriate topics for participants to talk about.

WHAT TO DO

Explain that listening skills often diminish in older adults. This can be because of depression, worry, preoccupation with health problems or diminished hearing. However, maintaining listening skills is vitally important as a means of communicating and staying connected with others and the outside world. It is therefore well worth looking at current listening skills and how they might be improved.

Ask participants what they think obstacles to good listening are. Write the comments on the whiteboard or flipchart. These might include:

- » Constantly interrupting when someone is trying to say something

- » Standing too close to the person

- » Monopolising the conversation with what interests you

- » Looking bored and disinterested

- » Avoiding eye contact

- » Not checking or indicating you understand what is being said

- » Sighing and looking at your watch

- » Using a disinterested tone of voice

Follow up by asking them what they think helps when listening to someone. These might include:

- » Keeping good eye contact

- » Leaning forward slightly to indicate interest

- » Asking open-ended questions

- » Making reassuring comments such as 'Go on...', 'Tell me more...', 'That's interesting...', 'I can understand that...'

» Showing concern and interest as appropriate in facial expressions

» Checking you understand what is being said

» Responding in an appropriate way

» Keeping appropriate physical distance

After discussion, split the group into subgroups of three people. Instruct one member of each subgroup to talk about a topic while someone else listens. The third person observes and makes notes, listing what the listener does well and what could be improved. After a few moments the observer then gives feedback. All observers then move to another subgroup, taking on a different role. The same process is followed again with a new observer and listener. Observers keep moving to another subgroup each time so that eventually everyone has talked about a topic, listened, been an observer and had feedback.

Finally, bring everyone back together as one group and invite comments. Ask if anyone has learned about any good and bad listening habits they have exhibited.

COMMENT

It helps to give people topics they can talk about each time, such as:

» Favourite meals, holidays, films

» Getting married

» Children's behaviour today

» Retiring

» Voting

» A hobby

» What makes them angry

» Modern technology

» Parenting

» A recent outing

LET'S TALK

PURPOSE

To help people get to know each other better and get them talking.

WHAT YOU'LL NEED

No materials required.

WHAT TO DO

Split the group into pairs and decide who is going to be A and who B. Now instruct the As that they will have two minutes to talk to their partner and tell them something about themselves. They can talk about anything they want to: a job they have done, a hobby, a holiday, their family, where they were born, where they live, what they have done during the past week, what films or books they like, for example. After two minutes stop the proceedings and instruct the Bs that they now have two minutes to talk to their partner, telling them something about themselves.

After both partners have held a conversation ask all the As to move on to another B partner and go through the same process again. Continue until everyone has had an opportunity to talk to everyone else. Encourage participants to choose different topics to talk about each time they change partners.

When completed, bring everyone back together and ask:

» Would anyone like to tell everyone about anything humorous, unusual or interesting (but not embarrassing) they have learned about one of their partners?

» Have you enjoyed the conversations?

» Have you got to know each other better?

» Would you normally take such a short time to get to know everyone? If not, why not?

COMMENT

If limited for time you can shorten the activity by reducing the number of partner changes.

SKETCHES

PURPOSE

To provide an alternative way to express feelings, ambitions or to elicit information about difficult topics.

WHAT YOU'LL NEED

Drawing paper, crayons and pencils.

WHAT TO DO

Hand out the drawing materials and ask participants to sketch two pictures. One drawing should show how they are feeling now and the second how they would like to feel in a set time in the future – a week, a month or a year. The sketches can be diagrammatic, abstract or of a scene that illustrates their feelings. Emphasise that the pictures do not have to be well drawn. A black blob may illustrate feeling depressed or a smiley face feeling happy.

When completed, ask everyone to show their drawings and interpret them for the group. Other group members can ask questions to aid understanding. Any issues that emerge will need to be appropriately addressed.

COMMENT

You can use this in a variety of ways to enable expression. For example:

» An ambition they had as a youth and an ambition now

» How they feel in the group and how they would like to feel

» Relationships with their family now and how they would like them to be

» Something they are angry about and something that pleases them

» A hobby they have done in the past and a hobby they would like to do now

You can make the subjects match the situations of individuals in the group.

SHOWING CONSIDERATION AND RESPECT

PURPOSE

To increase socialisation by showing consideration and respect to others.

WHAT YOU'LL NEED

A whiteboard or flipchart, a marker and some paper and pens or pencils. For the alternative you will require some large sheets of paper, a marker for each subgroup and some Blu Tack or similar to place the sheets on the wall.

WHAT TO DO

Explain that showing consideration and respect is an important part of enabling us to communicate well and build personal relationships. It helps us make friends, obtain help when we need it, enjoy companionship, get along with people we may not particularly like and prompts others to respect us.

Ask each person to reflect on their own behaviour and, in turn, state a way in which they have shown consideration and respect for other people in the past. This might be by:

> » Making an apology
>
> » Being tactful
>
> » Listening to some else's point of view
>
> » Complimenting someone else
>
> » Keeping appointments
>
> » Offering assistance
>
> » Respecting differences
>
> » Keeping a promise

Write the behaviours on a board or flipchart. Then, when everyone has contributed, invite group members to call out as many other behaviours which show good manners and respect as they can. Add these to the list on the board.

Give out some paper and pens or pencils and ask participants to reflect on their own behaviour and write down three ways in which they personally could show respect and consideration for others in their daily routine that they have been neglecting.

End the activity with everyone, in turn, stating one of the actions they are going to take to show consideration and respect to others.

COMMENT

Instead of writing a long list on the board (after each person states a way in which they have shown respect and consideration for others in the past), you could split the group members into two or three subgroups. Then give each subgroup a large sheet of paper and a marker pen and ask them to compile separate lists which they then place on a wall and present to the whole group.

IT'S THE WAY I SAY IT

PURPOSE

To encourage creative thinking and increase understanding of how to use body language as a way of communicating.

WHAT YOU'LL NEED

Pre-prepared slips of paper with a communication written on each and a bag, box or hat.

WHAT TO DO

Prepare a number of communications appropriate to group members written on slips of paper. Examples are:

> » I'm too hot
>
> » I'm cold
>
> » It's too noisy in here. I can't hear you.
>
> » My leg hurts
>
> » I feel nauseous
>
> » I need time to think
>
> » I'm happy here
>
> » Come with me to see the doctor
>
> » I want to go to sleep
>
> » I would like to see my grandchildren

Seat everyone in a circle and invite participants to choose a slip from the bag, box or hat. Each person then takes a turn in the middle of the circle and communicates what is written on their slip of paper using body language only.

When everyone has had a turn, lead a discussion on the difficulties of communicating and understanding body language. Ask questions such as:

> » Can you always tell what people mean by their expressions and gestures?
>
> » Do gestures and expressions have different meanings to different people?
>
> » Do people's expressions always match what they are saying when they speak?

» Do any group members use gestures and expressions to communicate words they can't remember or things they have difficulty communicating?

» What are the obstacles?

COMMENT

Because of some age-related loss of hearing, vision, memory and other cognitive abilities, practising using facial expressions, hand gestures, sign language and other non-verbal methods to convey meaning can become more important as one grows older.

SIMILES

PURPOSE

To enable expression of feeling, be creative, and have fun.

WHAT YOU'LL NEED

No materials required.

WHAT TO DO

Explain that a simile is a figure of speech that compares one thing with another and usually uses the words 'as' or 'like'. For example:

...as scared as a mouse

...as cold as ice

...like a fish out of water

...like a bird basking in the sun

Ask participants if they can think of a few other examples, then invite individuals to express how they feel by making up a simile using the word 'as' or 'like' involving a living creative such as an animal, a fish or a bird. Each person, in turn, states their simile beginning:

'I feel _____ (*as brave as a lion*).'

'I feel _____ (*like a bear with a sore head*).'

After a round, ask people if they would like to change their simile to one that someone else has used and which matches how they feel more accurately.

Next, have a round of people using a simile to state how they would like to feel. If they are happy with their previous simile they can restate it, or they can make up another.

End by talking about the similes chosen. Did anyone change them? Why? Did they feel any different after changing them?

COMMENT

Instead of using living creatures you could use similes involving flowers or vegetables.

OVERCOMING COMMUNICATION BARRIERS

PURPOSE

To enable individuals to identify ways of overcoming communication barriers.

WHAT YOU'LL NEED

Copies of the handout 'Overcoming Communication Barriers', paper and pens or pencils.

WHAT TO DO

Explain that the purpose of the activity is to identify ways of overcoming communication barriers. Then divide the group into pairs or subgroups of three of four people. Give each person a copy of the handout 'Overcoming Communication Barriers' and a pen or pencil. Tell the subgroups that they have fifteen minutes to discuss and come up with solutions to each of the problems listed.

After fifteen minutes invite each subgroup to give feedback on their ideas to the whole group. Identify the best solution for each problem and then ask, 'Why don't we do these things automatically?'

COMMENT

You can also ask participants if anyone has come across other obstacles to good communication and discuss ideas to overcome them.

HANDOUT: OVERCOMING COMMUNICATION BARRIERS

Barrier	Suggestions to make it easier to communicate
You or the person you are talking to is feeling very stressed.	
There is a lot of noise around you.	
The person does not appear to be listening or does not respond to what you are saying.	
The person has a strong accent.	
The person is speaking very slowly or softly.	

Barrier	Suggestions to make it easier to communicate
You, or the person you are speaking to, has a hearing impairment.	
The person keeps using jargon or technical words you don't understand.	
The person keeps standing uncomfortably close to you.	
The person keeps speaking too fast for you to understand.	
You, or the person, is too tired to concentrate.	
You, or the person, is very angry or emotionally upset.	
The person is sitting down or in a wheelchair and you are standing.	

MEMORY

ACTIVITIES TO HELP WITH MEMORY

CURRENT AFFAIRS

PURPOSE

To reinforce memory of what is happening in the world, and give the opportunity to express personal opinions and explore other viewpoints.

WHAT YOU'LL NEED

Articles cut from national or local newspapers about events or current issues.

WHAT TO DO

Give out the articles and invite participants to read them. After a set time invite one person to tell the group what their article was about. The group then discuss the issue and give their viewpoint on the topic. When this has been exhausted, invite someone else to tell the group what their article was about. This is then discussed. Continue in this manner until everyone has had an opportunity to present and discuss their article.

COMMENT

Instead of cutting out articles, give out newspapers and invite participants to scan them and pick out an article of interest. Then continue in the same manner as above. Repetition, by reading or watching events on TV and then talking about them, will help to reinforce memory and keep people up to date with current events.

THIS IS MY LIFE

PURPOSE

To maintain and improve mental capacity and help memory retention.

WHAT YOU'LL NEED

No particular materials unless you plan something special and, of course, tea and biscuits or cake.

WHAT TO DO

Invite participants, in turn, to share with the group what has been happening to them over the past week. They may have had a visit from a family member, gone on a trip, taken part in a craft activity, watched a movie, done some gardening, read a book, listened to music, visited the dentist or outpatients, painted a picture, written a letter or spoken to a grandchild in a different country using Skype.

Encourage other group members to ask questions about the experiences to help individuals enlarge and say how they felt about the events. They may have done very little or been bored doing something. Other participants can then make suggestions about different things they could do during the coming week. Do make sure that everyone gets an opportunity to talk about something that has happened to them or they have done.

COMMENT

Many older people lack the opportunity to talk to others about the current events in their lives and what they have been doing. Talking about and discussing these events will help to reinforce memory about events and what they have learned. You can also encourage, where possible, individuals to bring along something they have completed, such as a picture they have painted, a book they have read, a jumper they have knitted, or they can share pictures of places they have visited, visitors they have had. The group can be made into a natural social gathering with a break for tea and cakes which some of the members may have baked. Opportunities will also arise to mark special occasions such as birthdays or special trips.

GETTING ORGANISED

PURPOSE

To aid memory by introducing some organisation into individual lifestyles.

WHAT YOU'LL NEED

A whiteboard or flipchart, a marker, copies of the handout 'Getting Organised' and some pens.

WHAT TO DO

Introduce the activity by explaining that many instances of forgetting and losing things can be remedied by introducing some simple organisation methods. Many people already have systems which they have used throughout life. Some of these, because of changes in circumstances or health, may not work as effectively as they have in the past. Other people may never have felt the need to be organised and have managed fine up to now. Explain that when people do not have a system of keeping track of appointments, plans for the coming weeks, paying bills, remembering birthdays, keeping track of scissors, hearing aids or spectacles, phoning a friend, putting the rubbish out, and so on, they are more likely to be forgetful. It may therefore be helpful to develop a few organisational habits to help with memory. Though it takes some initial effort to form the habit, it saves time and frustration in the long run.

Having introduced the topic, ask people to call out some of the areas in which they sometimes experience difficulty or frustration. You can write a few of these on a whiteboard or flipchart. After a short discussion about memory difficulties give out the handout 'Getting Organised' and ask group members to complete the section 'Areas in which becoming more organised will help me remember are'. They can write down up to five areas. When completed, break participants into small subgroups of at least three people. Now ask each person to choose one of their memory problems and discuss it in their subgroup, come up with some possible solutions and write them down on their handout. Each person then chooses one of the suggested solutions to try.

Next, bring everyone back together as one group and invite each person to state the problem and solution they have chosen to use.

COMMENT

You can follow this up at the next group meeting by asking people how they are progressing, problems they have had putting the system into action and inviting them to choose another problem to work on. Avoid participants trying to establish more than one system at a time. Once one system is successfully established then move on to another problem. In this way, individuals can build on their successes and are more likely to carry out planned actions.

HANDOUT: GETTING ORGANISED

Areas in which becoming more organised will help me remember are:

1.

2.

3.

4.

5.

The area I want to organise first is:

Possible solutions are:

1.

2.

3.

The solution I will use is:

The area I want to organise next is:

Possible solutions are:

1.

2.

3.

The solution I will use is:

The area I want to organise next is:

Possible solutions are:

1.

2.

3.

The solution I will use is:

USING EXTERNAL REMINDERS

PURPOSE

To encourage the use of external reminders to aid memory.

WHAT YOU'LL NEED

Large sheets of paper and markers.

WHAT TO DO

Remind participants that most people use external reminders at all stages of life – not just when they are older. Examples are: keeping an appointments diary, either written or on a smartphone, making a shopping list, using an oven timer, or using a pillbox with compartments for each day of the week. Using these devices or written reminders means you don't have to worry about forgetting something. Using something in the environment as a cue leaves you free to think about other things. Point out that individuals may have used many of the techniques they are going to discuss but the activity may help them adapt and use them in different ways.

Split the participants into three subgroups and give them a large sheet of paper and a marker. Number the subgroups 1, 2 and 3. Instruct:

» Group 1 to discuss and list written reminders. Examples are:

- Writing a list of health questions to ask your doctor

- Keeping a list of names you want to remember, such as neighbours, members of a social group

- Recording birthdays and other dates you want to remember at the beginning of each year or keeping a birthday book

- Keeping a list of passwords in a secure place – for credit cards, online banking and smart devices, for example

» Group 2 to discuss and list auditory reminders. Examples are:

- Using a timer to remind you when to do something, for example when a meal is cooked, when to make a phone call

- If you are out and want to remember to do something when you get home, ringing home and leaving a message on your answering machine

- Carrying a small dictation machine; when something occurs to you that you want to remember, recording a message you can listen to later

- Using smartphone alarm settings to remind yourself to do something or to take medication

» Group 3 to discuss and list changing something in the environment as a reminder. Examples are:

- Putting items you want to take with you on an outing by the door

- Putting keys in the shoes you are going to wear to remind you to take them with you

- Having specific places to keep items so you always know where they are

- Using object cues. Putting your watch on the wrong wrist or the wrong way round, for example. Each time you look at it will bring to mind what you want to remember

After a set time, bring the participants back together. Each group, in turn, presents the different techniques they have discussed. Encourage all participants to add additional methods they use or have used.

Finish the activity by inviting each person, in turn, to state two techniques they will try before the next session.

COMMENT

It is always worth following this up in the next session by asking people how they have got on and discussing any problems they have encountered implementing their chosen techniques.

REMEMBER THIS...

PURPOSE

To challenge recall of old – and retention of new – memories.

WHAT YOU'LL NEED

A timer or watch.

WHAT TO DO

Set the timer for two or three minutes. Read out one of the questions/topics below or make up others appropriate to the group. Instruct the participants to close their eyes and think about the topic. Tell them to imagine that they are there observing the scene. What do they see, smell, hear, taste, touch and feel? After the allotted time participants open their eyes. Ask if they remembered more than they thought they would. Then invite volunteers, in turn, to relate the memory. Next, ask another question and go through the process again. You can either focus on long- or short-term memory, or alternate between the two.

» Who was your first love?

» What was your first job?

» What were your grandparents like?

» What was the first wedding you attended?

» What was the last school you attended like?

» Did you have a best friend at school?

» How did you spend your last birthday?

» What did you do last Sunday?

» What do you recall about your most recent holiday?

» What happened in the last episode of your favourite TV programme?

» What did you have to eat yesterday?

» What happened on your last outing to the shops?

COMMENT

Encourage group members to ask questions to prompt memories when individuals are relating their stories.

MEMORY CONCERNS

PURPOSE

To help establish individual memory worries and work out strategies to deal with them.

WHAT YOU'LL NEED

Copies of the handout 'Memory Concerns' and pens or pencils.

WHAT TO DO

Explain that learning several different memory techniques takes a lot of time and effort. This can be off-putting and can result in people not bothering to use any strategies. To sustain motivation we all need to choose methods that address our own particular memory difficulties. To do this we need to consider what these are but still remember to enjoy day-to-day living. This might include, for example, recalling birthdays, appointments, cooking instructions, recipes, directions from A to B, shopping items or how to open a tin.

Give out the handout 'Memory Concerns' and ask participants to list any difficulties they experience. These should be split into things they consider essential, important and other non-essential things they would like to remember better. They then decide which concern they would like to work on first, leaving the sections 'Suggestions how I might do this are' and 'I am going to do this by' blank.

When completed, invite individuals, in turn, to share the issue they are going to work on. Group members make suggestions on how they might do this. For example, for remembering appointments they might suggest keeping an appointments diary or calendar. The person writes the suggestions down and decides from these what they are going to do.

COMMENT

It is best to avoid individuals working on more than one or at the most two problems at a time, as this can be demotivating and result in the person giving up. Explain that once they have succeeded in overcoming one difficulty they can then tackle another. Also, making changes in habits and establishing new routines and making them habitual can take time. Handouts can be kept and followed up in a later group session with suggestions for tackling other identified problems.

HANDOUT: MEMORY CONCERNS

Things I would like to remember better are:

Essential things	Important things	Other things

Suggestions how I might do this are:

I am going to do this by:

What I would like to work on first is:

NAME THAT PERSON

PURPOSE

To increase observation skills, share and memorise names.

WHAT YOU'LL NEED

No materials required.

WHAT TO DO

Ask participants, in turn, to state their name and something about themselves. This might be 'My name is Nora and I write poetry'. When completed, instruct group members to have a good look at everyone else, then ask participants to stand up, one at a time, and face away from the group. Another person then describes a group member. The person standing up tries to name the person from the description. If they have difficulty, tell them the one thing the person from the description stated about themselves and see if that helps. You can also give other hints. Once the group member has been identified, the person guessing sits down and someone else has a turn. Continue in this way until everyone has participated.

End the activity by leading a discussion on methods individuals use to help them remember people's names. For example, repeating it several times, writing it down, envisioning the person doing something silly, rhyming it: 'Jolly Molly'. Ask how important they think it is to pay attention and be observant.

COMMENT

You can make this easier by having participants just guess the name of the person being described or having each person describe themselves. Hearing the voice will probably help spark the memory. Or make it more difficult by having each person state two things about themselves to be remembered.

WHAT DO YOU REMEMBER?

PURPOSE

To learn about each other and practise observation, listening and memory skills.

WHAT YOU'LL NEED

No materials required.

WHAT TO DO

Sit everyone in a circle. Instruct each person, in turn, to state their name and three things about themselves. Stress that members should pay close attention to what people say as they will need to remember it. When everyone has spoken, repeat the process but this time individuals don't talk about themselves but about another group member, saying their name and the three things that person originally stated.

End the activity by leading a discussion on methods people use to aid memory when being given information on a day-to-day basis. This might include making a note when on the telephone, or asking the doctor, nurse or receptionist to write things down.

COMMENT

Variations on this activity would be to have group members, in turn, state their name and three things about themselves. The person next to them then repeats what they said and states their own name and three things about him/herself. This is repeated until everyone has had a turn. To make it easier or more difficult for either variation you can decrease or increase the number of statements individuals make.

KIM'S GAME

PURPOSE

To exercise memory skills and learn strategies to aid memory.

WHAT YOU'LL NEED

10–15 items laid out on a tray, a cloth to cover it, paper and pens or pencils.

WHAT TO DO

Place the tray on a table so that everyone can see it clearly. Remove the cloth and ask everyone to make a mental note of all the items. Participants can walk around the tray to get a good view. After a couple of minutes cover the tray up again with the cloth. Next, give everyone a piece of paper and a pen or pencil and ask them to write down as many of the items as they can remember. When this has been completed, ask group members, in turn, to call out one item they have written down until all the items have been named.

Next, lead a discussion about the methods people used to help them remember items. Ask:

» Did they count the items?

» Did they classify them by size, shape, colour, or whether stationery or kitchen items, for example, or use other methods?

» Can similar methods be used to remember other things such as shopping? For example: vegetables, frozen foods, bakery, dairy produce.

Encourage people to express and share any memory difficulties and the methods they use to deal with them.

COMMENT

A popular game that is fun and enables people to learn memory skills from each other.

MENTAL WALK

PURPOSE

To practise a strategy to aid memory and have fun.

WHAT YOU'LL NEED

No materials required.

WHAT TO DO

Explain that to forget is normal for most of us. We are bombarded by so much information and detail that it is a healthy default to forget, unless, of course, there is something that we do want to remember. One method to help remember things is to go on a mental walk each day. To demonstrate, ask group members to think of one thing they did earlier in the day, such as going for a walk in the park, taking part in a group activity, getting up, having breakfast and getting ready to go out. Instruct them to sit quietly, close their eyes and, starting at the beginning, mentally visualise everything they did, saw, heard, smelled and tasted. After a few minutes ask for volunteers, in turn, to describe what they remembered. Then ask:

» Did you remember a lot more than you expected?

» In what situations could you use this method to help register details in the memory? (After listening to a talk, reading a section of a book, holding an important conversation, being given instructions, being introduced to new people, and so on.)

Point out that saying things out loud, telling them to someone else or writing them down will reinforce this further. Also, suggest that spending a few quiet moments each day going through the day's events will help reinforce memory of the important things they want to recall at a later time.

COMMENT

If individuals repeat the same mental walk though events several times at intervals, they are more likely to remember what they want at a later date. This is really good for memorising names.

AN EXPERIENCE TO REMEMBER

PURPOSE

To use experiences people have had during their lives to inspire creativity, and retain memory and the value of that memory.

WHAT YOU'LL NEED

A range of art materials including paper, watercolours, paint brushes, colouring pencils, drawing pencils.

WHAT TO DO

Discuss participants' past experiences. These might be recent, such as a visit to the museum, a birthday party, seeing a rainbow or seeing birds in the garden. It might be further in the past: a favourite place, a house they lived in, a trip abroad, a school playground or a place of work. Make sure each person has zoned in on a memory that stands out for them. Next, instruct participants to draw or paint the memory as best they can. It doesn't have to be a brilliant drawing. For example, they can use matchstick figures for men and women or bubbles for speech. They might also like to give the picture a title. When completed, invite each person to show and talk about their drawing or painting. End by asking them how they felt about doing the activity. Did it help refresh and bring the memory alive?

COMMENT

You can restrict the activity to a recent memory or choose a particular period, time in life or topic such as schooldays, teenage years, early adulthood, family life, a happy time.

SPIRITUALITY

ACTIVITIES FOCUSING ON SPIRITUAL WELLBEING

FEELING PRODUCTIVE

PURPOSE

To encourage individuals to engage in activities that they feel are productive and give meaning to life.

WHAT YOU'LL NEED

Copies of the handout 'Feeling Productive' and pens.

WHAT TO DO

Explain that throughout life we work at or do something which we feel is productive and meaningful to us. This can be making products, serving food in a restaurant, teaching or doing something like being a car mechanic that is useful and contributes to society in some way. Later in life, after retirement, we still need to be productive and do things which provide meaning – however small the projects might be or how old we are. These can be different things in different situations and at different times in life. For example:

> » Painting pictures

> » Putting together a family history

> » Singing in a choir

> » Sorting photos into albums as a record of events in a son's or daughter's life

> » Creating flower arrangements

> » Visiting a friend who is unable to get out

> » Making decorations for a grand-daughter's birthday

> » Knitting to raise money for charity

Ask participants for examples of things they have done in the past that gave them a feeling of being productive and a sense of meaning in life. Ask if there is any way they might continue to use their earlier skills in the present. For example, someone might have had a sense of satisfaction from befriending new work colleagues. Could they now use these skills as a volunteer in a local community or club of some sort?

After some discussion give out the handout 'Feeling Productive' and invite participants to complete the first section, 'I have felt productive in the past when'. When this has been filled in, split participants into pairs to discuss and help each other complete the remainder of the handout.

End the activity by bringing everyone back together and inviting volunteers to share what they are going to do, and when.

COMMENT

Over a lifetime, participants will have done quite a number of jobs and activities they have enjoyed and which were meaningful to them.

HANDOUT: FEELING PRODUCTIVE

I have felt productive in the past when:

1.

2.

3.

4.

I could use the skills acquired doing the above now by:

Steps I could take to do this are:

1.

2.

3.

4.

I will take step 1 on:

WHAT IS IMPORTANT IN LIFE

PURPOSE

To clarify what is important, raise awareness about beliefs and maintain a sense of self.

WHAT YOU'LL NEED

Pens or pencils and paper.

WHAT TO DO

Give out paper and pens or pencils. Explain that you want everyone to draw their own coat of arms. First, everyone draws a shield and divides it into four sections. Then in each section they draw an item that represents something important to them. This might be:

» Someone doing something, to indicate work

» Two people shaking hands or embracing, to show friendship

» A family group, to indicate family

» Someone assisting someone ill or disabled, to indicate caring for others

» A church, to indicate worship

» A pile of money, to indicate wealth

They can also use words or phrases on the drawing if they wish. When everyone has completed their coat of arms invite them, in turn, to show their drawing and talk briefly about what it means.

COMMENT

You can vary this activity by getting participants to draw four things which are important to them:

» In their social life

» In daily life

» In their spiritual life

» As a member of the community

» In the group

» Within the family

In the struggle of day-to-day living people frequently lose sight of what is important to them, resulting in feelings of discontent and lack of sense of purpose.

MY VALUES AND BELIEFS

PURPOSE

To remind individuals about their core values, clarify what they mean to them and how they are currently being honoured in their life.

WHAT YOU'LL NEED

Copies of the handout 'My Values and Beliefs', pens, a marker and a whiteboard or flipchart.

WHAT TO DO

Explain that when values and beliefs are known and honoured then we feel contented, happy and motivated. If we dishonour our values then we can feel unhappy, discontented, stressed and uneasy. Our values also influence how we react, are motivated and behave in different situations. This makes it important to maintain awareness of our core values, bearing in mind that these may change at different times of life.

Invite participants to give some examples of values and beliefs and write these on a whiteboard or flipchart. These might include:

» Being honest	» Being true to my religion or culture	» Having a willingness to explore
» Looking after my health	» Being open-minded	» Being flexible
» Having fun	» Showing appreciation	» Being there for family
» Being creative	» Respecting others	» Inspiring others
» Staying connected		

Now pick out a value or belief and ask: 'What does this value mean to you?' If you have chosen 'Looking after my health', a response from the person who volunteered it might be 'having a sense of wellbeing' or 'keeping fit'. Do this at least twice.

Next, give out some pens and the handout 'My Values and Beliefs', and ask participants to fill it in using up to eight values and beliefs which are important to them – but, not to just copy them from the board.

When everyone has completed the task, invite participants, in turn, to share the value they feel is not being sufficiently honoured and the things they could do to honour it.

COMMENT

If anyone has difficulty identifying core values, ask them:

>> What are you doing when you feel most content? What values or beliefs are you being true to?

>> Looking back on life, when did you feel most content? What were you doing? What core values were being fulfilled at that time?

>> When you are 100 years old or so and look back, what would you like to be most proud about? What core values would be fulfilled?

If individuals struggle with completing the handout, it can be useful to have participants work in pairs – particularly when working on the 'Things which I can do to honour this value are' section.

HANDOUT: MY VALUES AND BELIEFS

Core values and beliefs	What this value/belief means to me is:	On a scale of 0–10 rate how much this value is being honoured currently in your life (0 represents never and 10 represents all the time):
1.		
2.		
3.		
4.		
5.		
6.		
7.		
8.		

A value which is not being sufficiently honoured in my life is:

Things which I can do to honour this value are:

1.

2.

3.

4.

INSIDE AND OUTSIDE

PURPOSE

To raise awareness of the outer and inner aspects of self.

WHAT YOU'LL NEED

Boxes, a range of paints, colouring pencils, markers, art materials, magazines, decorative paper, scissors and glue.

WHAT TO DO

Give each person a box (shoe boxes work well) and instruct them to decorate it, both inside and outside, using any materials they wish, drawing, painting, colouring, symbols, writing, using decorative paper or using words and pictures cut from the magazines.

The outside of the box should represent their outer self – the part of them that they present to other people. This might be cheerfulness, always busy, hobbies or things they do, skills, being efficient, being independent and so on. The inside of the box should represent their inner self – their hopes, ambitions, fears, doubts, beliefs and things which are important to them such as listening to or playing music, being creative, going to a place of worship, helping others. Music symbols can be used to represent music, a book to represent reading, and so on.

When completed, invite volunteers to show their box and talk briefly about what the various colours, pictures and symbols represent. Make it very clear that individuals may choose to show or disclose little or nothing about the interior of the box, though it is important that they are aware of its content.

COMMENT

Omitting boxes, this activity works equally well using two sheets of paper, one headed 'Inside' and the other 'Outside', and asking participants to draw, using colour, pictures, symbols, words, and so on. The boxes, however, do provide additional novelty.

IMPROVING MIND AND SPIRIT

PURPOSE

To explore ways of improving spiritual wellbeing by enabling people to connect with activities they find meaningful and which provide them with the strength to face the challenges of life.

WHAT YOU'LL NEED

A whiteboard or flipchart and marker.

WHAT TO DO

Lead a discussion on what participants understand by the term 'spiritual life'. Some may identify it with their religion or culture, others with doing creative activities such as art, sport or craft, having time for themselves, being at one with nature, the pleasure they derive from a hobby, enjoying friendship and good company, helping others, and so on. Questions you could ask to explore the theme and as prompts are:

- » What sort of things do you do to relax?
- » Do you have favourite books you return to again and again?
- » What is your ideal holiday?
- » What has been most important to you in the past?
- » Do you enjoy nature?
- » Do you prefer any particular time of the year?
- » Do you feel there is any purpose to life?

Point out that we often focus attention on our physical wellbeing and neglect this mind and spirit aspect of life. Now ask participants what sort of things we can all do to improve our spiritual wellbeing and keep a balance in life. Write the suggestions on the board. These might include things like: listening to favourite music, birdwatching, treating others with kindness, being non-judgemental and open-minded, meeting friends for coffee and a chat, working as a volunteer, or creating a regular time for quiet reflection.

When a good long list has been produced, ask participants to think about and state, in turn, two things they could do which would benefit their mind and spirit.

COMMENT

Across different cultures and religions, people nurture their minds and spirits in many different ways. Very basically, this activity addresses spirituality as connecting with things which individuals find meaningful, enriching their lives.

LIFE FOCUS

PURPOSE

To reflect on what has been the main focus in life so far and how this may influence future choices.

WHAT YOU'LL NEED

Copies of the handout 'Life Focus' and pens or pencils.

WHAT TO DO

Point out that just as our bodies physically change as we age and mature, so do our values and focus in life. Give out the handout 'Life Focus'. Ask participants to think back to the different periods in their life and tick the things which were important to them in that period. They should use the blank spaces to list other things which are not included.

When completed, lead a discussion. Ask:

» Which focuses or values do they consider to have had the greatest influence on their lives so far – for good or bad?

» How has it influenced them?

» Has any focus or theme continued throughout their life so far?

» What have proved to be their greatest strengths?

» What will influence their choices in the future?

End the activity by inviting each person, in turn, to state one focus from the past which will influence their choices in the future.

COMMENT

This is an activity which can throw up many surprises for individuals and give them greater self-awareness and understanding.

HANDOUT: LIFE FOCUS

Focus	Childhood	Early adulthood	Later adulthood	Retirement +
Helping other people				
Music				
Having goals				
Feeling secure				
Family life				
Having a hobby				
A sense of belonging				
Competitions				
Work				
Possessions				
A good social life				
Having my own space				
Family get-togethers				
Meditation				
Having a challenge				
Money				

Focus	Childhood	Early adulthood	Later adulthood	Retirement +
Learning				
Religion				
Friendships				
Structure				
Time on my own				
Interacting with nature				
Keeping fit				
Romance				
Gardening				
Raising children				

CONNECTING WITH NATURE

PURPOSE

To encourage individuals to maintain spiritual awareness though a connection with nature

WHAT YOU'LL NEED

A whiteboard or flipchart and a marker.

WHAT TO DO

Explain that people connect with nature in different ways throughout life. They may do this through gardening, walking in the park, keeping animals, swimming in the sea, climbing, and so on. Now ask participants:

» How have they enjoyed keeping in contact with nature throughout life? (Write a list of suggestions on the whiteboard or flipchart.)

» How did doing that affect how they felt?

» Did it help them relax or feel at one with nature?

Next, ask how people – bearing in mind their current environment – could keep in touch with nature. This might include:

» Birdwatching from a window

» Watching the stars at night

» Watching nature change through the seasons

» Watching TV programmes about nature

» Keeping dried leaves in books

» Pressing flowers

» Creating collages using leaves and flowers

» Planting flowers or vegetables

» Walking or sitting by the sea or a river

» Collecting pine cones

» Drawing scenes or animals

» Keeping a diary of observations about nature

» Visiting garden centres

» Listen to recordings of birds or sea sounds

Write the suggestions on the whiteboard or flipchart. End by asking participants in turn to choose one of the suggestions they would like to do, and how and when they will do it.

COMMENT

Activities that enable people to connect with nature have amazing results. They provide enjoyment, enable them to relax and have an enormous impact on their spiritual and physical wellbeing.

A GUIDE FROM THE PAST

PURPOSE

To receive guidance and reassurance from people who have supported individuals in the past.

WHAT YOU'LL NEED

No materials required.

WHAT TO DO

State that throughout life participants will have had mentors, people who have advised, supported, guided or helped them in some way. Such people will have had their best interests at heart. They might have been a teacher, a friend, a partner, a priest, a parent or grandparent, a work colleague or supervisor. Point out that it is likely that participants have had different mentors at different times and in different areas of life. Some of these people might be deceased or might not currently be in contact with them.

Now invite participants to think of one of these mentors from the past – picture them in their imagination. Tell them to bear in mind the things they gave guidance about (work, personal life, children, a hobby, for example) and ask them a question: 'What can I do about...?' Now listen for their answer. What would they tell you? Can you hear their voice?

Allow a moment or two for people to focus, and then ask:

- » Did you hear the person speak to you?

- » How did that make you feel?

- » What advice did they give you?

- » How do you feel about using this process when you need advice, reassurance or when you feel alone with a problem?

COMMENT

You may find that some group members already do this. Point out that it is important that people use this process to reach out to people who have had a positive influence on them and not those who criticised or have been negative. It is also a way of knowing that, even though some of the people they reach out to might have passed away, they are not alone in life.

SOCIAL COMMUNICATION

ACTIVITIES PURELY FOR FUN, ENJOYMENT AND SOCIALISING

A PERFECT DAY

PURPOSE

To cheer everyone up and help raise spirits when feeling down.

WHAT YOU'LL NEED

Pens and paper.

WHAT TO DO

1. Ask participants to think for a moment and recall a perfect day from the past. This might be their wedding day, a day they went shopping with a friend, a family outing, a day on their own in the garden or a day they went swimming in the sea. Each person, in turn, relates their happy day. Encourage group members to ask questions and help individuals expand on their experience. Ensure that they include as much information as possible: what they had for breakfast, what they did in the morning, had for lunch, activities in the afternoon and evening, and so on.

2. Invite everyone to think about what would make a perfect day for them in the near future – perhaps in one or two weeks' time. After a few moments for thought invite individuals, in turn, to share their idea of a perfect day. Again, have them include as much information as possible. Encourage them to think of some special things they would like to do. Examples might include: visit a special place, go for a walk in the forest or have a favourite meal.

3. Have a general discussion about how the perfect days could be made possible. Could some participants make it happen themselves? What would be needed for others to have their special day?

COMMENT

Make notes about each person's idea of a perfect day and arrange for some of the things mentioned to happen. Ideal for a birthday! You can also use this as a writing activity by getting them to write about their perfect day in the past and then invite them to share the details. Do the same for a future perfect day.

PET HATES

PURPOSE

To stimulate discussion and encourage expression about things which annoy and irritate.

WHAT YOU'LL NEED

Pens and some paper for participants to make notes of what is said by their partner.

WHAT TO DO

Split the group into pairs and instruct each person in turn to talk to their partner about at least two things which they find annoying or irritating. These might include:

» Vandalism	» Insects	» Noisy eaters
» Gossip	» Hot weather	» People who mumble
» Smokers	» Badly behaved children	» Breaking a nail
» Rudeness	» Bossiness	» Constipation
» Non-stop talkers	» Celebrities	» Bullies
» Selfishness	» Cold weather	» Cramps

After a set time, five or ten minutes, bring everyone back into a circle and instruct each person to present their partner's two pet hates. 'Margery's pet hates are gossips and cramps. She hates gossips because...'

COMMENT

If you allow pet hates to include people, stipulate that it is restricted to famous people and does not include anyone in the group or who is known personally to group members. You can also encourage other group members to comment or ask questions about each pet hate.

MUSICAL GAMES

PURPOSE

To encourage people to mix, communicate with others and have fun.

WHAT YOU'LL NEED

A number of paper and pencil games, board games, quizzes or crossword puzzles with which group members are familiar or which are easy to do. You can allot the same game to each pair or use a mix. Examples of games are: Hangman, Snakes and Ladders, Draughts, Scrabble. Pens and paper as required.

WHAT TO DO

Divide the group into pairs and get them to sit two on each table – the tables having been arranged in a circle, square or straight line with the necessary equipment for the appropriate game. Explain that on the word 'go', or when the music starts, each pair starts playing the game. After a set period, say ten minutes, or when the music stops, each player moves to the table on their left and continues with the game on that table with a different person. Continue in this fashion until everyone has played with each other at least twice.

COMMENT

You might need to hover in the background to explain game rules to those who have forgotten the rules or how to play. To include gentle exercise you could use games that entail movement, such as darts, indoor bowls, marbles or tiddlywinks. These work well if you have sufficient space.

EARTH, AIR, FIRE AND WATER

PURPOSE

To increase mental alertness and develop flexibility of thinking.

WHAT YOU'LL NEED

No materials needed.

WHAT TO DO

Arrange the participants in a circle and ask for a volunteer to sit in the middle. This person then points to a person in the circle and calls out one of the categories: *Earth, Air, Fire* or *Water.* That person then responds as appropriate:

Earth: the name of an animal that lives on the earth

Air: the name of a bird that flies through the air

Fire: a piece of equipment, material or substance used to help fight fire

Water: a type of fish that lives in water

If the person responding has difficulty thinking of something, other group members can help by giving clues. When the appropriate response has been given, the person in the centre then points to someone else and calls out another category. Once an animal, bird or fish has been named it should not be repeated. The activity continues in this manner as long as people keep coming up with appropriate responses.

COMMENT

You can change the person in the middle so everyone gets a turn. Also, instead of having someone in the middle you can start the activity by calling someone by name, stating a category and throwing a soft ball or bean bag to them. The game then continues in this fashion for as long as possible.

MAKING CONNECTIONS

PURPOSE

To enable participants to get to know each other better and make connections with others.

WHAT YOU'LL NEED

You will need to have asked participants to bring two or three photographs involving other people – family members, friends or acquaintances. These might be of an outing to the seaside or a football match, a wedding anniversary, a holiday, in a yoga class, a romantic occasion. Small-group photographs work well. Participants might like some paper and a pen to make notes as an aid to memory.

WHAT TO DO

Instruct group members to find a partner and talk to one another about their pictures, explaining who is in the photograph, the relationship and significance to them, and where and when they were taken. Individuals can make notes to aid memory.

After a set time, have everyone reassemble and invite each participant to present his or her partner to the group, using the partner's photographs. Encourage them to highlight new things they have discovered about one another and what they have in common.

End the activity by discussing with the group whether they have learned any surprising new facts about their partners or their connections with other people.

COMMENT

Even when people know each other well, new information and connections usually emerge.

INFORMATION SHARE

PURPOSE

To help people get to know each better and create an environment in which everyone can socialise freely.

WHAT YOU'LL NEED

Copies of the handout 'Information Share' and pens.

WHAT TO DO

Introduce the activity as a way for individuals to share information and get to know each other better. Give out the handout 'Information Share' and tell the group they have ten or fifteen minutes to work out the answers. It is helpful to give a reminder when time is running out.

Bring everyone back together as a group. Invite participants, in turn, to share the information they have found out about different members of the group. Encourage other group members to ask questions of the person the information is about. For example: 'How long did you live in France? How did you cope with the language?'

COMMENT

You can use more or fewer questions on the questionnaire, depending on how long you want the activity to last. You can also change the activities and questions listed to suit group member backgrounds.

HANDOUT: INFORMATION SHARE

Move around the room, talk to other group members, find people who have done any of the following. Write their names and their answers to the questions in the appropriate sections. Talk to as many people as possible and find someone who:

Has lived in a foreign country. Which country?

Plays a musical instrument. Which instrument?

Enjoys reading. Do they have a favourite book?

Has kept animals. Which animals?

Has or had an unusual collection. What did or do they collect?

Has a hobby such as writing poetry, painting, gardening.

Loves singing. What types of songs?

Enjoys the theatre. Do they have a favourite play or musical?

Plays or has played a sport. Which sport?

Watches TV soaps. Which is their favourite?

WHO IS IT?

PURPOSE

To help group members get to know each other better and sharpen intuitive ability.

WHAT YOU'LL NEED

Some small cards and pens.

WHAT TO DO

Give everyone a card and a pen. Ask each person to write on the card something about himself or herself that no one in the group would know. Provide examples such as: 'I had a short part in the film *Gone with the Wind*', 'When I was ten I broke my arm ice-skating', 'I have always wanted to be a pilot', 'I have a tattoo of John Lennon on my left shoulder'.

When the task has been completed, collect, shuffle and redistribute the cards. If anyone gets their own card they must keep it secret. Now ask participants, in turn, to read out what is written on their card. The other group members try to guess who has written the statement. When the writer has been found out, encourage the person to elaborate on the statement and group members to ask questions about it.

End the activity by discussing what clues people used to match the disclosure to the person who wrote it. Point out that picking up on these types of clues is a good starting point to making connections with others.

COMMENT

You can have the group repeat the activity, sharing new information.

SECRETS

PURPOSE

To energise group members, instil a sense of fun, change the mood of the group, enable people get to know each other better and break down barriers.

WHAT YOU'LL NEED

No materials needed.

WHAT TO DO

Jokingly, ask if people have any dark secrets in their past. Give an example of your own: 'I broke a favourite ornament my mother prized that belonged to her grandmother. I told her the cat knocked it over. She never ever queried it and I've never confessed. I still feel really bad about it.' Now ask people to pair up with someone they know least well in the group. The pair share a secret that no one knows about them. Next, invite individuals to state their partner's name and divulge their secret to the group. 'This is John. When he first started work he...' Continue in this manner until everyone has had a turn.

COMMENT

This activity introduces a sense of fun and enjoyment when group members are feeling down and you want to lift the mood of the group.

LISTS

PURPOSE

Lists can be made to serve whatever purpose you want: for fun, to build confidence and self-esteem, to broach difficult topics, to discuss spiritual issues or for reminiscence.

WHAT YOU'LL NEED

Pens and paper.

WHAT TO DO

Give out pens and paper and ask participants to write down ten things on a particular topic. Choose one of the examples below or make up an appropriate topic yourself.

- » 10 ways I can look after myself
- » 10 things I'm good at
- » 10 things I like about myself
- » 10 things I've enjoyed doing
- » 10 sacrifices I've made
- » 10 things I value in life
- » 10 things I believe in
- » 10 skills I have acquired
- » 10 pieces of advice I would like to give my children
- » 10 things I expect from myself
- » 10 fears I have about giving up control
- » 10 memories from my past
- » 10 lessons I have learned
- » 10 things that make me laugh
- » 10 things I'm sad about
- » 10 things I like about me

When the lists are complete, invite participants to share and discuss their lists.

COMMENT

You can, of course, alter the number of things people write down to suit the time available. Also, create titles for fun or to broach issues for group members.

FAVOURITE THINGS

PURPOSE

To break down barriers and help participants get to know each other better.

WHAT YOU'LL NEED

No materials required.

WHAT TO DO

Ask each person, in turn, to state a favourite thing and why they like it. They may not have an absolute favourite but can give the first thought that comes to mind. Here are some suggestions you can use:

» Sport	» Time of life	» Actor or actress
» A lucky number	» Colour	» TV show
» Taste	» Animal	» Time of day
» Hobby	» City	» Book or magazine
» Flower	» Country	» Drink
» Singer	» Meal	» Piece of clothing to wear
» Time of year	» Game	» Job
» Film	» Subject at school	» Mode of travel

COMMENT

You can do two or three rounds of favourite things, or you can alternate with rounds of least favourite things.

WRITING

ACTIVITIES USING WRITING FOR HEALTH AND WELLBEING

MEMORY STIMULATION

PURPOSE

To use the senses to stimulate memories.

WHAT YOU'LL NEED

Objects which are not necessarily easily identified by touch, such as a feather, a piece of material, sea shells, a candle, small ornaments, small wooden carvings, a piece of wallpaper, textured boxes, a bracelet, a furry toy animal, a framed photo, a notebook. (Avoid practical everyday things such as cups, saucers or pens which are easily identified and tend to be less effective in stimulating imagination. Also ensure the objects are fairly robust and won't fall apart when handled.) Pens and paper.

WHAT TO DO

Ask individuals to sit with their hands in their laps and close their eyes. Explain that you'll be placing an object in their hands – nothing nasty, creepy or unpleasant. Tell them to feel, smell, shake or knock the object gently against something. They can use any of the senses to explore it – except sight. While they are doing this, ask the group questions:

» What does your object feel like?

» What colour do you think it is?

» What might it be used for?

» How old is it?

» Is it natural or man-made?

» Who might it belong to?

» Does it remind you of something – a memory, a person, an event, an experience or an emotion?

Allow people to ponder on their objects for a few minutes and then tell them you are going to take them away. When you have done this, ask them to open their eyes and to start writing about any memories the objects have recalled. Allow a pre-set time. Ten minutes is usually sufficient.

When the time is up, invite each person, in turn, to read out what they have written and afterwards show everyone the object they held.

COMMENT

If anyone feels uncomfortable about closing their eyes, say they can keep them open if they wish. You can also do this exercise omitting the writing. Instead, invite each person, in turn, to talk about any memories stimulated.

UNSENT LETTERS

PURPOSE

To enable expression of emotion, opinions, deepest feelings, resentments, affections, hostilities and controversial points of view in a safe atmosphere.

WHAT YOU'LL NEED

Paper and pens.

WHAT TO DO

Explain that you want everyone to write a letter which will not be sent or seen by anyone. It will be destroyed. The letter can be to anyone. This might be to:

» A friend who has died or moved and they never have had the chance to tell them something

» Someone who has upset them

» A daughter or son who has not been in touch for some time

» A partner who has left them, died or caused them pain

» Express anger about something that has happened in the past

» Acknowledge feelings about inadequacy as a parent

» Explain disappointment or regret about something

» State how much they miss someone

State that participants can write about feelings, hostilities, emotions present and past, anger, grief, resentments, affections or controversial opinions. Because no one is going to see what they write they can express themselves, using whatever language they want, without fear of anyone knowing what they wish to say. This enables them to gain closure and gain insight about feelings.

After a set time writing about a chosen issue, ask them how they feel now that they have been able to express their feelings in writing. Don't forget to ask people to then destroy the letter. They can be ripped up or passed through a paper shredder.

COMMENT

Unsent letters can be about anyone or anything, alive, dead, an organisation, an institute, beliefs or to someone famous. Letters may start with expressions such as, 'What I want to say is...' or 'I want you to know...' It is important that individuals do not censure their feelings but let them out. Writing and destroying a letter conveys a discharge of feelings and enables the person to express personal issues, come to terms with them and move on.

WITH THESE HANDS

PURPOSE

To tell life stories using different parts of the body.

WHAT YOU'LL NEED

Paper and pens.

WHAT TO DO

Explain that we live in our bodies and experience the world through the different parts of them using the senses – sight, hearing, touch, smell and taste. Ask participants to look at and examine their hands. How do they feel about them? How have they used them over the years? What sort of things have they done with them? Baked cakes, made jewellery, created a garden, played the piano, painted and decorated houses, assembled cars, played cards, stolen things, made sculptures, and so on. After some brief discussion to get people thinking, invite participants to focus on one aspect, incident or situation in which their hands have played a major role. They can write a poem or just tell a story about their hands. Here is the start of a short example:

> *I love these hands; they have helped me earn my living all my life. They are short, stubby and quite ugly but always strong and dependable. Many times they have gotten me out of trouble. The first time was in 1953 after I got my first job. I was working on some high scaffolding when a lorry crashed into it knocking a platform away from under my feet. Luckily my hands grabbed a cross bar...*

When participants have finished writing, invite volunteers to read out their work

COMMENT

You can also do this activity using other parts of the body such as feet, eyes, hair, shoulders, teeth, ears and nose. You may like to give participants a choice of which body part viewpoint they wish to write about. The activity can also be done verbally, giving participants time to think and then inviting them to relate their story.

ABOUT ME

PURPOSE

To explore identity, personal contradictions and encourage self-acceptance.

WHAT YOU'LL NEED

Pens and paper.

WHAT TO DO

Ask participants to write down at least five one-sentence statements about themselves. These can be about good or bad characteristics: likes, dislikes, fears, ambitions, hopes or dreams. Request that at least one statement contains a contradiction about themselves. Here are some example sentences:

I like to take my time doing things

I am always late but get angry when other people are not on time

I fear losing my independence

I love going to the theatre

I am indecisive but become impatient when others won't make up their minds

I have a vivid imagination

I find it difficult to trust people but get offended when other people don't trust me

I love cats

I enjoy helping others

I like to keep myself to myself but I'm lonely

Now invite them to choose one or two of these statements to write about in more detail. They can give examples from their life illustrating the statement or write a poem or verse about it. When a set time is up, invite participants to read theirs out.

COMMENT

This activity also works when done verbally. First, get participants to write down a statement about themselves and then invite them to read it out and talk about it briefly. Encourage other group members to ask questions to help them discuss it. It is often the character contradictions that are the most interesting and fun.

DEAR FUTURE ME

PURPOSE

To explore hopes and fears about the future.

WHAT YOU'LL NEED

Pen, paper and envelopes.

WHAT TO DO

Explain that we are forever making decisions on behalf of who we will become in the future. We agree or feel obliged to go along with different courses of action. What can you tell your future self about it? What do you want for your future self? What are your hopes, fears and advice for them? Will your future self have regrets or celebrations for what you are doing now?

Here is a sample letter written to a future self:

Dear Future Me,

At the moment I feel miserable and upset. And you are the cause. It's you I'm thinking about. I've just sold my lovely house and moved into this small flat. It's very nice and there is someone on hand if you need help. But it doesn't have the memories. There are so many memories both happy and sad I don't want to forget. Will they now fade? Do you still remember? I want to write down some of these memories. Have you done it? Is there some sort of record to show my grandchildren? Have you included pictures so they can remember their Grandad who died so suddenly last year?

I've always been scared of the future, forgetting to enjoy the here and now. I hope you've stopped doing that. Enjoy being 85. It's not so bad really, is it? Of course, you have aches and pains, high blood pressure, find stairs difficult and take even more tablets. What did you expect? I'm afraid to ask some questions. Is my best friend Julia still around?

I'm having a hard time adjusting right now. But I can see it's in my power to make life better for you. I hope I haven't let you down. I'm doing my best, so don't hate me too much.

Do something nice for your birthday. Celebrate. I bet the family will all be round later. Have a drink on me.

Me

When participants are clear about the process, ask them to write a future letter to themselves. Select an appropriate time period or let them choose. This could be in six months, one, five or ten years' time.

End the activity by asking participants how they feel now after having written their letter to their future self. Provide opportunity for individuals who would like to share their letter to do so by reading them out.

COMMENT

Of course, this writing activity can be completed using email instead of letter format and printed off to reflect on at a later date. Alternatively, participants can actually send an email to themselves to be received in the future. To do this they will need to go to www.futureme.org.

WRITING SPRINGBOARDS

PURPOSE

To aid reflection on past, present, future, what is happening now, feelings, and so on.

WHAT YOU'LL NEED

Pens, paper, a marker, and a whiteboard or flipchart.

WHAT TO DO

Write a springboard opening statement on a whiteboard or flipchart for group members to write about. Alternatively, write three or four and ask participants to choose one to write about. Make it clear they can write in any format they wish, for example straight narrative or a poem. Examples of opening statements are:

Five things I want to do (today, tomorrow, this week, this year, etc.) are...

What I most value in my life is...

I'm proud of myself for...

I feel (sad, happy, angry, indecisive, excited, etc.) because...

What worries me most about (today, tomorrow, the future, the journey, the upcoming event, the visit, etc.) is...

The happiest time of my life was...

What I feel right now is...

I believe that...

What gives me hope for the future is...

My biggest (secret, fear, hope, regret, wish, worry, love, etc.) is...

What I value most in relationships is...

The most important thing for me to do is...

When participants have finished writing, invite volunteers to read theirs out. Make it clear that those who do not wish to read out do not need to do so.

COMMENT

These opening gambits can be worded to aid reflection and expression of feelings about most things and to build self-esteem.

CLUSTERING

PURPOSE

To help participants generate ideas, make new associations, break internal barriers and unblock thoughts and ideas.

WHAT YOU'LL NEED

Pens and paper.

WHAT TO DO

Provide participants with a starting point by asking them to write a word or phrase in the middle of a clean sheet of paper. This might be a word or phrase which describes:

>> Their current mood

>> Something that is worrying them

>> Something they have got to do

>> An important date

>> Someone's name

>> A significant place

>> A fear

They then draw a ring round this word or phrase. Next they write the first related thought that comes to mind, circle it and connect it to the first circle. They continue in this way until they reach the edge of the page. They then return to the centre and start again. They do this three or four times or until the page is filled. Each person then chooses one circled word or phrase that stands out to them and writes freely about this for 5–10 minutes.

Participants may or may not wish to read theirs out. If not, end by asking them how they now feel. Has the exercise opened up any new trains of thought?

COMMENT

Alternatively, instead of choosing a single word or phrase to write about, have them look at all the associations they have made and ask themselves what stands out. Is there a pattern of thought or feeling? They then write about this.

CONFLICTS

PURPOSE

To help with making decisions, look at unfinished business, express and come to terms with difficult situations, change or modify behaviour.

WHAT YOU'LL NEED

Pens and paper.

WHAT TO DO

Explain that life is full of conflicts. Learning to cope with them is essential to survival. This may include:

- » Inner conflict (repressed urges, temptation, our personal code, loyalty or guilt)

- » Nature (ageing, disease, the weather, time or the sea)

- » The social aspects of life (politics, morality, obligation, financial situations, customs, the law)

- » Objects (machines, clothes, tools, traffic, furniture)

- » Living things (other people, animals, birds, insects)

- » The supernatural (fate, superstition, God, the devil, good, evil, magic, myth, taboos)

Now ask each person to choose a conflict in their life and imagine they are stuck in a lift with someone. This can be anyone living, dead or from fiction. The person might be a role model, someone admired, a friend or a relative. Next they imagine having a conversation with them about the conflict and write the dialogue. The dialogue might begin something like:

Peter: *I want to ask you how you cope with growing older. I am on my own now. My wife died two years ago and my son Jason lives abroad. I feel so alone. You kept going when Dad died and continued to enjoy life.*

Mother: *Yes, I did continue to enjoy some things. But it was hard, especially at first. Just like you're finding it now. Keeping in touch with old friends and making new ones was a tremendous help.*

Peter: *I understand that but you always had loads of friends. I find it difficult making the effort to do anything. What's the point?*

Mother: *You sound depressed. If things are that bad you should see the doctor. What about your Amateur Dramatics? You gave it up because you were looking after your wife, Jane. Couldn't you join the local group again?*

And so on.

After a period of writing, ask if anyone is surprised by what they have written. Has it given them a different perspective? Some people may like to read theirs out but, as the topics chosen and the words written are private, do make it clear that this is optional.

COMMENT

When responding to material read out, avoid being judgemental or commenting in a critical way on structure or style. Try to gauge what the reader wants in response and ask for clarification of anything in a gentle manner. Also, some people may find this writing exercise difficult at first, but it is worth persevering.

INFLUENCES

PURPOSE

To evaluate the factors which have influenced and continue to influence individuals.

WHAT YOU'LL NEED

Pens, paper, a whiteboard or flipchart and a marker pen.

WHAT TO DO

Explain that we are all born in different circumstances within different countries, cultures and social groupings. Economic circumstances, gender, educational opportunities, religion or marriage may affect what we do and how we live. These may help or constrict opportunities. Also, perhaps because of improvement in economic circumstances or moving from one country to another, our attitudes and values may change.

Initiate a very brief discussion about things which have influenced or changed individuals' lives and values. Write a list on the whiteboard or flipchart. This might include:

» Places	» Religion	» A friend	» A job
» Culture	» Marriage	» A mentor	» A teacher
» Gender	» Social class	» Education	» An experience
» A relation		» Travelling	

When the list has been completed, ask individuals to write about things that have influenced and changed their lives. Suggest they think about:

» The way in which they have been influenced or changed – for better or worse

» How this might influence their choices in the future

» If there has been a negative impact, how it might be possible to now make further changes to improve things

After writing, give opportunity for reading out and discussion. Ask if anyone has had any insights of which they had not previously been aware. What do individuals think has had the greatest influence on them?

COMMENT

This is a good exercise to help individuals obtain a balanced view of what has influenced and continues to influence their decisions.

GRATITUDE LETTERS

PURPOSE

To build confidence and self-esteem and create a feel-good mood.

WHAT YOU'LL NEED

Pens and paper.

WHAT TO DO

Ask participants to imagine a familiar person writing them a letter of gratitude. This might be someone they have known in the past or currently. It could be someone they have worked with, supported, cared for, taught something, mentored and helped in some way. It might just be something small they have done for the person or cause. Instruct them to outline all the things for which the person would be grateful, writing it from that person's perspective.

When complete, invite each person, in turn, to read their letter out. Group members can contribute anything not mentioned for which they think the viewpoint person might be grateful.

COMMENT

A feel-good and uplifting exercise. Encourage people to keep their letter and read it aloud to themselves when they are alone and feeling down.

REMAINING ACTIVE

ACTIVITIES TO ENCOURAGE PHYSICAL MOVEMENT

MIME

PURPOSE

To communicate without using words, identify and respond to imagined objects and use gentle movement.

WHAT YOU'LL NEED

A list of objects and actions to use in case participants have difficulty thinking of one.

WHAT TO DO

1. Start by doing a demonstration mime using an object. This might be putting on lipstick, playing the piano or tying your shoelaces. Group members guess what you are doing.

2. Call out an action and instruct everyone to mime it together. Ask participants to imagine the objects they are using. Help them by saying things like: 'What kind of seeds are you planting? What do they feel like?' Do this several times.

3. When people feel comfortable miming, ask individuals, in turn, to think of an object and action and mime it. The other group members guess what the mime represents. If anyone has difficulty thinking of a mime you can whisper one in their ear or give them a slip of paper with a mime written on it.

4. You can follow this up by dividing the group into pairs and getting them to work together to work out a mime which they can do together. Examples might be: making a bed, loading a truck, hanging wallpaper, washing and drying dishes, playing cricket, hoisting a sail. Once each pair have worked out their mime, get them to take turns presenting it. The other group members guess what they are doing.

COMMENT

Different mimes can be chosen depending on the abilities of participants. Examples are:

» From a seated position: reading a newspaper, arranging flowers, stringing beads, threading a needle, playing cards, cooking an omelette, writing a letter

» Standing: walking a dog, mixing a cake and putting it in the oven, plastering a wall, cleaning the car, planting a shrub, playing golf, bowling, cutting the hedge

You can also stop the activity at any of the stages or choose just to do one of them.

BALL GAME

PURPOSE

To provide gentle exercise and enjoyment, and maintain reflexes.

WHAT YOU'LL NEED

A large soft ball and chairs.

WHAT TO DO

Arrange the chairs in a circle. Call out a participant's name and gently throw the ball to that person. That person then takes control of the ball, calls out someone else's name and throws the ball to them. After everyone has caught the ball a few times, stop the proceedings. This time call out someone's name and kick the ball gently to them. They then call out someone else's name and kick the ball to them. This continues until everyone has participated.

COMMENT

This is also a good activity to help any new members of a group learn everyone's name.

FUN EXERCISE

PURPOSE

To exercise the body, help participants relax and have fun.

WHAT YOU'LL NEED

No materials needed.

WHAT TO DO

This activity can be performed seated or standing. Do make sure that participants are far enough apart so they can spread their arms horizontal to the floor without touching anyone else. You then call out directions whilst demonstrating an exercise. They can be gentle or more demanding, to suit the abilities of group members. Simple directions might include:

Move your head gently from side to side

Drop your chin to your chest and slowly rotate your head in a circle

Move your shoulders up and down and around and around

Bend your arms at the elbow and swing your hands back and forwards

Rotate your hands in a circle from the wrist

Wiggle your fingers

Rotate your upper torso, first to the left and then to the right

Rotate your hips in a circular motion

Lift your knees, first the left and then the right

Lift one foot and flex it forward from the ankle and then upwards a few times, then do the same using the other ankle

Using the ankle, rotate each foot in turn

Wiggle your toes

COMMENT

You can add to the difficulty and fun of this by adapting it to a version of the old children's game of 'Simon Says'. For example, you call out the direction 'Simon says put your hands on your head' or 'Simon says wiggle your fingers', and everyone carries out the action. If you call out a command but do not preface it with 'Simon Says' and someone does the action, then that person takes over calling out the commands. This makes the activity good for quick thinking and concentration. It increases the fun element and brings smiles to faces. It is also a good activity to lighten the atmosphere or give a lift to a group that is heavy going.

OBSTACLE COURSE

PURPOSE

To help participants relax, have fun and exercise the body.

WHAT YOU'LL NEED

A list of set tasks and whatever is required to complete them. When compiling the list be sure to take into account the abilities and safety of the participants.

WHAT TO DO

Create a succession of obstacles or tasks for participants to do to test their physical skills and abilities. The less able can be escorted round the course. Obstacles and tasks might include:

- » Stepping over a box
- » Walking five paces with a book balanced on the head
- » Throwing a ball or bean bag into a waste basket from three metres away
- » Carrying a jug of water three metres
- » Miming the name of a film, TV show or book to someone
- » Doing a funny walk
- » Going under a rope at shoulder height
- » Juggling or pretending to juggle three balls for one minute
- » Running or walking on the spot for one minute
- » Walking a figure of eight drawn on the floor twice

Make the obstacles and tasks suit the abilities of participants.

COMMENT

How you facilitate this can vary. You can do it as an obstacle course, or alternatively, write a list of tasks on a whiteboard or flipchart and get group members, in turn, to call out someone's name and instruct them to do one of the tasks. No one should be asked to do the same task twice.

WALK THIS WAY

PURPOSE

To have fun, inspire creativity and exercise.

WHAT YOU'LL NEED

No materials required.

WHAT TO DO

Ask people to clear away any chairs so there are no obstacles in the centre of the room. Next, call out a type of animal, insect, fish, bird or person. For example, a drunk, a cowboy, a fashion model, a truck driver, an English gent, a swaggering youth, a geisha girl, the Pope, an elephant, a giraffe, a monkey, a tiger, a spider, a duck, a cow, a swan, a shark. All group members then move around the room mimicking how they imagine the named type of being would walk or more. Every minute or so, call out a different type for participants to mimic. Continue in this manner for ten or fifteen minutes or until participants begin to tire.

COMMENT

A variation would be to ask group members, in turn, to call out different types of person, animal, fish, and so on.

WHAT'S THIS?

PURPOSE

To encourage creativity and have fun while encouraging movement.

WHAT YOU'LL NEED

No materials required.

WHAT TO DO

Participants can stand or sit while doing this exercise. Each person takes a turn at drawing a huge fruit, animal, vegetable or object in the air using their hands and arms. Before drawing, they state the type of thing it is. For example, a fruit, a building, transport, a country or an animal. Grapes might be the outline shape of a hanging bunch with a number of smaller circles drawn close together inside the shape. A bus might be the outline shape with two circles for wheels on the bottom line. The other group members guess what has been drawn in the air and then everyone repeats the action, drawing the item in unison. Continue in this manner until everyone in the group has had a turn drawing a few times.

COMMENT

You can restrict the drawing to just a single type of thing such as fruit, or change this as soon as everybody has had a turn at drawing the chosen object. But, when deciding, do bear in mind the abilities of group members. This activity is particularly good for arm exercise.

MOVING TO THE RHYTHM OF THE MUSIC

PURPOSE

To encourage movement, aid relaxation and have fun.

WHAT YOU'LL NEED

Scarves, flags, bunting, short cane sticks or scarf-sized pieces of material, a range of different music recordings – both fast and slow – and a music player.

WHAT TO DO

Give each person a scarf, bunting, and so on. Arrange participants in a circle and stand in the middle. Alternatively have them spread out, making sure everyone can see you; or you could have them in two lines facing each other. Participants can do this activity sitting or standing. Do make sure they are far enough apart that they don't interfere with each other's movements. Start the music and lead everyone by example in moving to the rhythm. Everyone can do their own thing, swirling a scarf, conducting the music, or, if standing, move their body as well as swirling a scarf to the beat.

It is best to begin with a slow rhythm and then alternate between fast and slow tracks. End with a slow track. Also vary the music, as tastes will differ.

COMMENT

You can use themes in different sessions. Themes could include: a period such as the 1970s, Country and Western, music from popular films, Indian music. Be aware of the abilities of your group members and what they can do. The more enthusiastic you are and the more fun you make it, the more enjoyable it will be.

MIRROR ON THE WALL

PURPOSE

To aid concentration, exercise the body and have fun.

WHAT YOU'LL NEED

No materials needed.

WHAT TO DO

Ask participants to imagine they have just got up and are looking at themselves in a full-length mirror. You are the reflection they see. Ask them all to follow your movements. Start by yawning, leaning your head to the right, then the left, stretching your arms up in the air. Do movements such as putting your tongue out, wrinkling your nose, brushing your teeth, pointing your toes, one leg at a time, and so on. Go on to perform other movements such as:

» Shaving

» Washing your face

» Putting on make-up

» Getting dressed

» Eating breakfast

» Washing the dishes

» Cleaning the windows

» Vacuuming the lounge

» Peeling potatoes

» Baking a cake

Perform the actions in an exaggerated manner and at a pace group members can keep up with. If necessary, or to make it easier, you can call out the action you are about to do.

COMMENT

You can invite group members, in turn, to take over being the mirror. The others then follow their movements. Participants can do this activity either sitting or standing. Make sure the movements to be mirrored are appropriate to participants' abilities.

BUILDING CONFIDENCE

ACTIVITIES TO HELP RETAIN
CONFIDENCE AND
A POSITIVE SELF-IMAGE

POSITIVE NOTES

PURPOSE

To improve self-esteem.

WHAT YOU'LL NEED

Pens, and a stack of paper slips or small cards. Also, prepare an envelope or box for each participant with their name written on it.

WHAT TO DO

Ask each person to write something positive about each of the other members of the group on separate slips of paper. This can be something they like about them, a good quality or skill they have, a compliment about how they dress, and so on. Stress that it must be a positive statement. Examples are:

I do like your sense of humour.

You have a beautiful smile.

You are a good conversationalist.

I admire your sense of dress.

You are a good friend.

The slips of paper are then posted in the appropriate envelopes for each person which have been hung on a wall or placed around the room. When completed, hand out the envelopes to the appropriate people and give them time to read the notes. Next, have a discussion. Ask:

- » How did it feel when reading the notes?
- » How did it feel writing the complimentary notes?
- » How important is it to give and receive compliments every day?
- » How often do you do this when with friends, family or other people?

COMMENT

This activity works best with people who know each other. You can also get people to write the complimentary notes at the beginning of a group session, do other activities such as craft, and then get participants to read the notes at the end of the session. This makes sure everyone leaves the group feeling good.

WHAT MAKES ME FEEL GOOD?

PURPOSE

To help people identify what undermines confidence and what makes them feel good about themselves.

WHAT YOU'LL NEED

A whiteboard or flipchart, a marker, pens and paper.

WHAT TO DO

Ask group members to think about all the negative things they tell themselves or other people have told them and invite them to share these. Write them on a flipchart or whiteboard under the headings 'Other people told me' and 'Things I tell myself'. Examples might be:

Other people told me	Things I tell myself
'That's not for people like you'	'I'm not good enough'
'Anyone could have done that'	'Not at my age'
'You won't change at your time of life'	'I'm just a grandmother'
'You're useless'	'I could never do that'

When everyone has contributed to the lists, discuss how people react to these negative statements and thoughts. Do they take them to heart and permit them to make them feel bad? Or, should they challenge them and refuse to allow them to dictate their feelings?

Next, give each person a sheet of paper and a pen and instruct them to write down the heading 'I feel good about myself when...' Underneath they should list at least five things that make them feel good about themselves. Examples might be:

I feel good about myself when...

1. *I remind myself about what I have achieved.*

2. *I complete a drawing.*

3. *I sing along with my favourite pop stars.*

4. *I recall the lovely times I have had with my grand-daughter.*

5. *I have a chat and a laugh with friends over a cup of tea.*

6. *I read a good book.*

When completed, invite group members, one at a time, to call out one item from their list. End by suggesting that each day in the coming week they do one of the things that make them feel good.

COMMENT

Often very simple things can lift our moods when feeling down. But we forget to use them to help us feel better and more confident.

ACHIEVEMENTS

PURPOSE

To encourage participants to look back with pride and gain confidence from past achievements.

WHAT YOU'LL NEED

A whiteboard or flipchart and a marker.

WHAT TO DO

Ask participants a question or ask them to say something about their past achievements and write it on a whiteboard or flipchart. Briefly discuss the scope of the subject to prompt memories. Give participants a moment to reflect on the topic and then, in turn, invite them to share their achievements. Here are some typical questions and topics with introduction ideas to help participants recall their achievements.

» What has been your outstanding talent in life?

Have you been a good provider, fun to be with, a great organiser, good with money or a great cook? Perhaps you have been a peacemaker, the driving force, the main family support, the creative one, the innovator or the person who sees things through? How have you managed to achieve this and keep it going? Give examples of what you did and how you did it.

» Describe something you have done to help someone else.

Did you help someone through a difficult time, give advice or befriend someone you didn't like? Have you looked after someone who was ill or a dependent relative, helped a neighbour or done a voluntary job? Describe what you did and how it felt. How do you feel about it now?

» Describe a proud moment in your life.

What was it? What led up to it? Why did you do it? Was anyone else involved? How did you feel? How did you feel afterwards?

» What has been the most difficult thing in life for you to overcome?

Were you ill at some time? Have you ever encountered prejudice? Have you had a weight problem? Have you struggled with a bad temper? Did you, at some time, lack confidence or self-esteem? How were you affected and how did you overcome it?

» What has been the most satisfying experience in life for you?

Were you happy with your job, your children, married life or something you accomplished? Did you look after your parents or ensure your children had good opportunities in life?

» What do you consider your greatest accomplishment so far?

This may be an award, having a child, raising money for charity, something you were honoured with in public, a challenge you overcame, coping with a difficult situation, writing a book, or a contribution to your family or society. Did you do it alone or with a group of people?

» What have you done that might help generations to follow?

You may have helped to develop a sense of morality or pride in some people, helped with research, contributed in some way towards overcoming world poverty or disease, helped preserve historical buildings or helped someone learn a skill.

» What is the biggest compliment you have been paid?

Who made it? What did you do to warrant the compliment? Why did you do it? Was anyone else involved? Did it take a big effort on your part? Did the compliment surprise you? How did you feel then? How do you feel about it now?

When individuals are describing their achievements, ask other participants to encourage them by asking questions.

COMMENT

You can vary this activity. Write the different questions or requests on separate pieces of paper and have participants randomly pick one out of a bag or box. These are also good subjects to get people to write about.

MY QUALITIES

PURPOSE

To enable individuals to identify a quality about themselves and to translate the trait into positive attributes.

WHAT YOU'LL NEED

A foam or soft ball.

WHAT TO DO

Toss or bounce the ball to someone in the group. This person states their name and a quality about him/herself, something he/she does or anything about their life. For example:

'My name is John. I am a good cook.'

'I am Joan. I am very cautious about doing new things.'

The rest of the group respond 'That's a good quality', and the person then states the benefits or advantages of the quality or what it means to them or other people. For example:

'My cooking skills have meant my children formed healthy eating habits. I also earned a living from cooking.'

'Being cautious means that I always prepare well for anything I do and ensure risks are minimised.'

The individual then throws the ball to someone else. Continue in this manner until everyone has had an opportunity to state at least one of their qualities.

COMMENT

You can, of course, continue the process until everyone has stated two or three qualities they possess. Also, if anyone has difficulty translating their quality into benefits, get the other participants to ask questions to help them or point out benefits of the quality.

BEING POSITIVE

PURPOSE

To teach a technique that helps people translate negative thinking into positive behaviour and action.

WHAT YOU'LL NEED

A whiteboard or flipchart, a marker, pens and paper.

WHAT TO DO

Explain to participants that it is really worth taking time to tune into their thoughts and check out how they are thinking and describing things to themselves. Focusing on the negative in how we think and talk to ourselves makes it more difficult to get through the day while remaining realistically optimistic. Often thoughts run along the lines:

» I don't want any hassle tomorrow.

» I don't want to go shopping today.

» I don't want to spend any more money.

Thinking in these terms, focusing on the negative, makes it more difficult to achieve these goals. Even if you change 'I don't want...' to 'I want...' the statement will still contain hidden negatives such as the words 'lose' and 'stop':

» I want to lose weight.

» I want to stop spending money.

It is better to translate your thoughts and thinking into words which describe realistic positive behaviour and action. For example:

Thoughts normally used	Realistic positive behaviour and action
I don't want any hassle tomorrow	I will arrange a hassle-free day tomorrow
I want to stop spending money	I will reduce my spending each week by £10

It is important that the new statements are kept realistic. There is no point in anyone setting themselves up to fail by being unrealistic.

Write the examples on a whiteboard or flipchart and then ask participants for a few examples of thoughts or statements they use in daily life which are not expressed in terms of positive behaviour and action. Write these on the board and then invite participants to work in pairs, choosing two statements or thoughts of their own and restating them in terms of behaviour and action. They can write these down if it helps them to remember. When this has been completed, bring everyone back together and invite volunteers to share both their original statement and the new statement. End by asking how they feel about the new thoughts. Does it change how they feel about the issue in any way?

COMMENT

Thinking in terms of behaviour and action makes this a good activity to help motivate individuals into achieving both small and large tasks they want to do. However, do make sure they take it one step at a time and are realistic.

GRATITUDE

PURPOSE

To help change perspective, lift mood, be aware of the good things in life and be more optimistic.

WHAT YOU'LL NEED

Pens and paper.

WHAT TO DO

Give out some pens and paper and ask each participant to write down five things for which they are grateful in life. This might include good health, a supportive family, a good neighbour, enjoyment of a hobby, good eyesight, being able to see the funny side of things or having a reliable friend. When completed, invite everyone, in turn, to read out the things for which they feel grateful.

COMMENT

This can be varied. If the group meets late in the morning or in the afternoon ask them what they feel grateful for on that day, which might include having had a good breakfast, enjoying the sunshine, having someone to talk to, a hug from a grandchild, enjoying sitting in the park looking at the flowers, the smell of cooking, a phone call, coming to the group. This is an activity you can repeat on a regular basis and which trains people to be constantly aware of the good things, no matter how minor they seem.

POSITIVE HANDS

PURPOSE

To build feelings of goodwill and friendship and build confidence and self-esteem.

WHAT YOU'LL NEED

Sheets of paper and pencils or pens.

WHAT TO DO

Briefly discuss with participants how people feel when someone compliments or praises them. It not only makes the recipient of the praise feel better, but the person giving the praise also feels good. Divide the group into pairs. Give everyone a sheet of paper and a pen or pencil and ask them to write their name on the top of the sheet. Partners then trace a silhouette of the hand (either hand) of the person named.

When completed, regroup in a circle. Participants then pass their sheet of paper to the person on their left. That person then writes a compliment or something positive about the person named on the sheet. For example: 'Jane has good taste', 'Paul is good at drawing cartoons', 'Emma is kind'. Participants keep passing the hand silhouettes to their left until everyone has written a different compliment on each hand and the sheet is back in possession of the owner. Allow a moment or two for everyone to read and absorb what has been written about them and then ask them how they now feel. Are they surprised by any of the comments?

COMMENT

You might also like to ask participants how they now feel about other group members. Has anything changed?

MAINTAINING SELF-ESTEEM

PURPOSE

To boost self-esteem and help participants recognise and change self-defeating behaviours.

WHAT YOU'LL NEED

Large sheets of paper and markers. If doing the alternative below, a whiteboard or flipchart and a marker.

WHAT TO DO

Explain the difference between behaviours that boost self-esteem and those which are self-defeating by giving some examples. Behaviours which increase self-esteem might include: ringing a friend for a chat, having a new hair style, attending a hobby group, or doing voluntary work. Self-defeating behaviours might be: thinking you are not important, not asking for help when you need it, or not eating properly.

When the concept is clear, split participants into two groups. Give each subgroup a large sheet of paper and a marker. Instruct one group to make a list of behaviours which increase self-esteem and the other to list behaviours which undermine self-esteem.

After a set time, have each subgroup present their lists. Discuss each item, why it is good or bad for self-esteem, and the effect the behaviour has on how individuals feel and their health. Invite group members to add to each other's lists.

End by asking each participant, in turn, to state a behaviour they will do to help boost their self-esteem and one they will stop doing that erodes their self-esteem.

COMMENT

An alternative to dividing the group into subgroups would be to brainstorm the two lists on a whiteboard.

CONFIDENCE MESSAGES

PURPOSE

To encourage participants to build confidence by sending positive messages to themselves.

WHAT YOU'LL NEED

Some sheets of paper and pens or pencils.

WHAT TO DO

Explain that the messages – negative and positive – we receive both about ourselves and from others can have a big impact on us. Constantly receiving or giving yourself negative messages erodes confidence. Receiving positive messages can have a significant effect on maintaining your confidence and giving you the emotional support you need to help you through a difficult time.

Give out some sheets of paper and ask participants to write their name on the top. Now ask participants to exchange sheets with someone else. That person writes down a list of qualities and strengths they see in the person named on the sheet. This might include things like: determined, efficient, hardworking, strong-minded, has overcome many difficulties in the past, good at problem solving. When completed, that person gives the sheet back to the owner who then adds additional strengths and qualities she/he knows they possess.

Complete the activity by inviting participants, in turn, to share their list of positive messages. Other group members may like to add additional strengths they have seen in the person. Finish by suggesting that individuals keep their lists of strengths and look at them from time to time, particularly when they are going through moments of doubt and uncertainty.

COMMENT

Self-doubt and uncertainty trouble all of us from time to time – even champions. Point out that the seven times Wimbledon tennis champion, Pete Sampras, has said that during a difficult period in his career he often carried a letter from his wife with him on to the court to help him through moments of self-doubt. The letter reminded him that he was a multiple champion and that he was possibly the best player to pick up a tennis racket.

HOW DO YOU SEE YOURSELF?

PURPOSE

To check individuals' self-perception against how others see them, how they would like to be seen and which things are most meaningful to them.

WHAT YOU'LL NEED

Copies of the handout 'How Do You See Yourself?' and pens or pencils.

WHAT TO DO

Give out the handout 'How Do You See Yourself?' and ask participants to complete it. They might think that other people see them as being 'efficient', 'a bit stand-offish' and 'honest'. Their ideal self might be as 'a good friend', 'supportive' and 'fun'. Things they have been praised or complimented for might be 'helping others', 'being a great cook' and 'being a hard worker'.

When everyone has completed the handout, invite each person, in turn, to read theirs out. Encourage other group members to comment on how accurate the person is on how they think others see them, how close they are to their ideal self, and add other praises and compliments. The person ends by stating which of the praises and compliments means the most to them.

COMMENT

Checking how people imagine other people see them against how they would like to be seen is not something people do very often. It can provide some pleasant surprises and give indications of some changes they might like to make. It is sometimes helpful to discuss this at the end of the activity.

HANDOUT: HOW DO YOU SEE YOURSELF?

Write three words or phrases that describe how you think other people see you.

1.

2.

3.

Write three words or phrases that describe your ideal self.

1.

2.

3.

Write down three things for which you have often been praised or complimented.

1.

2.

3.

Which of these compliments mean the most to you?

RESPONDING TO SITUATIONS

PURPOSE

To explore ways of responding to situations to give a more positive outcome.

WHAT YOU'LL NEED

Copies of the handout 'Responding to Situations' and pens or pencils.

WHAT TO DO

Explain that we all react to situations in different ways. At one end of the spectrum, one person's immediate reaction might be negative, interpreting events in a pessimistic way. Their immediate response is to look on the black side and view the situation in a bleak way. Thus problems often appear unsurmountable and disastrous. At the other end, a different person may see the situation as a challenge, a momentary blip that can be overcome or as a source for new opportunities. Point out that how we respond has an enormous impact on how we deal with everyday situations and how we feel.

To explore how participants respond, give out the handout 'Responding to Situations' and ask them to write down their immediate thoughts about the situations listed. When completed, split participants into pairs or small groups of three people. Now instruct them to work together and go through each of the answers that tend to be negative, discussing how the situation might be interpreted in a more positive light and therefore result in them dealing with it in a more satisfactory way.

End the activity by bringing everyone back together, inviting a few people to share their examples and asking how they feel about giving this a try when faced with situations in real life.

COMMENT

You can change the situations in the handout to make them more relevant to group members.

HANDOUT: RESPONDING TO SITUATIONS

Write down what your immediate thought would be if you were faced with the following situations.

1. You are complimented on a difficult task you have just completed.

    Your first thought: . . . .

2. A friend has barely spoken to you on an outing.

    Your first thought: . . . .

3. You have been asked to do something you don't like doing by a family member or friend.

    Your first thought: . . . .

4. You receive a letter from the police.

    Your first thought: . . . .

5. You receive an invitation to be presented with an honouree position.

    Your first thought: . . . .

6. Nobody has phoned, texted or emailed you for a few days.

    Your first thought: . . . .

7. Your son/daughter has not been in touch for a few weeks.

    Your first thought: . . . .

8. After working in the garden you feel a bit dizzy and sweaty.

    Your first thought: . . . .

REMINISCENCE

ACTIVITIES TO AID REMINISCENCE

MEMORIES IN A BAG

PURPOSE

To stimulate impromptu memories, help group members get to know each other better and form bonds.

WHAT YOU'LL NEED

Statements and/or questions written on slips of paper, and a bag.

WHAT TO DO

Sit everyone in a circle. Pass the bag around and ask everyone to take a slip of paper from it. If anyone doesn't like their question, allow them to pick another to replace it. Examples of statements and questions are:

> » Describe a typical day in your life when you were fifteen.
>
> » What have been your favourite radio or TV shows from the past?
>
> » What ambitions did you have as a teenager?
>
> » Talk about something you regret not doing.
>
> » Describe a happy time in your life.
>
> » Who did you feel closest to in your family?
>
> » Describe a typical day in your life at forty.
>
> » Talk about someone who has been a good friend. How did you meet?

Give people time to think and then get them, in turn, to follow the instructions on their slip of paper. Encourage other group members to ask questions to help individuals tell their story. If working with a large group, it is best to set a time limit of, say, one or two minutes for each person to talk.

COMMENT

You can use statements and questions covering life in general or set them around a specific time of life or topic such as childhood, teenage years, working life, adult life or social life. Instead of getting people to respond verbally, you could get them to write about their statement/question. After writing for five or ten minutes you might invite them to read out their responses.

MUSICAL MEMORIES

PURPOSE

To provide an opportunity to relax, enjoy music and reminisce.

WHAT YOU'LL NEED

A CD player and a collection of recordings from the past, appropriate to the age of group members.

WHAT TO DO

Play a chosen popular recording. Afterwards invite participants to comment. Ask what they were doing when the song or music was popular. Were they in love, married? Did they have children? What work were they doing? Where did they live? What are their memories of the period? After discussion, play another recording and invite more comments.

COMMENT

You can, of course, ask participants to bring along their favourite recordings from the past or prepare well in advance by asking them what their favourite recordings are and acquiring them. If individuals are able to, you can invite them to dance to the music. Another alternative is to choose a particular decade and play music from that time. You could, in a series of sessions, cover the lifetime of participants.

TIME OF LIFE

PURPOSE

To use age, as people have grown and matured, as a means of remembering past events.

WHAT YOU'LL NEED

Photographs cut from magazines of children, teenagers and adults at different stages of maturity.

WHAT TO DO

Distribute pictures of children playing, for example at the zoo or on the beach, to everyone. When they have had a few minutes to look and comment, ask them what memories they have of when they were that age. Do they remember similar outings? What were their favourite games? Do they remember doing things with their grandparents? What were they like? And so on.

In another session you might distribute pictures of teenagers. Again, ask age-appropriate questions. Did you have any teenage romances? Do you remember your first date? How did you cope with school and exams? Were you allocated jobs to do at home? What was your first job?

Yet again you can follow the same process with photographs of people in early adulthood or with young families. Then with middle-aged people, then when coming up to retirement and, lastly, when more mature after retirement. Always keep the questions appropriate to the age you are covering.

COMMENT

You could ask participants to bring along photographs of themselves as a child, a teenager and at different stages of adulthood. You can usually cover the whole of an individual's life in this way. You can also use the pictures as stimulus to encourage people to write about themselves at different ages.

RAISING A FAMILY

PURPOSE

To explore similarities and differences in raising children over three generations and how this has influenced individual lives.

WHAT YOU'LL NEED

If doing the improvisation, a whiteboard or flipchart and marker.

WHAT TO DO

Discuss the principles about how members of the group were raised. Were there any disagreements between their mothers and fathers and grandparents? What constraints, punishments and rewards were imposed on them? How has this affected their lives? After this has been explored, move on to how group members raised their children. Did they do it differently? What punishments, constraints and rewards did they impose? In what way? What effect did this have? Did they have any disagreements with their partners? Next, move on to how children are raised today. How does it differ from their day?

COMMENT

You could make a list on a whiteboard, as the discussion progresses, of some of the most troublesome problems in bringing up children and the approaches that were tried. You could then break the participants into subgroups. Give each subgroup one of the problems and get them, in turn, to improvise and act out short scenes based on the solution discussed.

NOTABLE EVENTS

PURPOSE

To remember events from the past, what effect they had on life, and compare the past with the present.

WHAT YOU'LL NEED

Place reproduced headlines from the past around the room on desks or walls to set the tone and get people talking. These could include events such as:

U.S. Pilot Shot Down Over Soviet Airspace

First Ever Spacewalk

I.R.A. Bomb Kills Mountbatten

Falklands War Breaks Out

Cleveland School Massacre

Berlin Wall Pulled Down

Princess Diana Killed in High-Speed Crash

Coalition Forces Invade Iraq

WHAT TO DO

Encourage group members to share memories evoked by the headlines. Ask questions such as:

» What was the general reaction of people at the time?

» How did you feel about it?

» What was happening in your life?

» Did it have any effect on you?

» What were people's main concerns at the time?

» Would there be the same reaction today?

» Do you feel any different about it today than you did then?

» What similar events have there been during your lifetime?

Encourage discussion about other similar events remembered by participants.

COMMENT

You might want to either cover one decade or the lifetime of participants. You can also stick to notable scandals or have headlines around past issues in your local area.

POWERFUL PLACES

PURPOSE

To use places to access memories and reflect on past experiences.

WHAT YOU'LL NEED

Pens and paper.

WHAT TO DO

Ask participants to think about a place in the past in which they felt safe. Give a few minutes for reflection and then invite group members, in turn, to describe the place, how old they were, what they were doing and how they felt. How do they feel now, looking back? Encourage other group members to ask questions about the place and what was happening at the time.

COMMENT

Other place topics you can use include places where they felt angry, trapped, loved, happy, sad, confused, independent, scared or excited. Alternatively, you can write three of four of these topics on a board or flipchart and invite people to choose their own topic. These also provide good subjects to get people to write about.

SMELLS IN MY LIFE

PURPOSE

To use sense of smell to access memories, reflect on past experiences and relate aromas to life moods.

WHAT YOU'LL NEED

Copies of the handout 'Smells in My Life', or whiteboard or flipchart and a marker. You might also be able to obtain and have available some typical smells which are safe to display or pass around, such as Bovril, lavender or baby powder.

WHAT TO DO

Either give out the handout or, alternatively, ask people to call out smells, scents or aromas they recall from different times in their life. Write these up on the whiteboard or flipchart. Ask participants:

» Do any smells evoke strong memories? What do they associate with them? A scene, an event, a person, a place?

Now ask group members to choose a smell that evokes a memory and, in turn, describe it. Encourage group members to ask questions about the memory – what, where, when, who, how – to help the person describe it fully.
   Finish the activity by asking:

» Which scents are comforting? Why?

» Which make people feel good?

» How could individuals use the smells that are comforting and make them feel good to help lift their mood when they feel down?

COMMENT

You can get participants to write about a memory associated with a smell rather than talk about it. You might also be able to obtain and have available many of the smells listed on the handout. If you can, ask participants to circulate and smell the different aromas before talking or writing about them.

HANDOUT: SMELLS IN MY LIFE

Freshly mown grass	Jasmine
Baby powder	Tea tree oil
Vicks vapour	Plasticine
Candyfloss	Candles
Cocoa butter	Perfume
Bonfires	Fish and chips
Chalk	Talcum powder
Pipe smoke	Musty garden shed
Chicken soup	Hairspray
Doughnuts	Savlon/Germolene
Cinnamon	Peppermint
Bovril	Popcorn
Muscle rub cream	Lavender
Leather (shoes)	Marker pens
Petrol	Roses
Coal tar soap	Old Spice
Baking	Barbecues
Salty scent of sea air	Creosote on fence panels
Pine	Furniture polish
Bubble gum	Bleach

MY LIFE IN A BAG

PURPOSE

To encourage people to value their individuality and their experience in life.

WHAT YOU'LL NEED

Prime participants by giving them a bag to bring five objects along to the group. These must say something about them and their past life. Examples are:

» A qualification certificate

» An ornament

» A piece of jewellery

» A photo showing a family group, a pet, friends, a holiday, a house or a garden

» A favourite children's book

» A piece of clothing that evokes a special memory

» A card received for a special occasion

» A theatre programme

» A travel souvenir

» An old work tool

Make sure that everyone is aware that they will be invited to show their chosen objects to the rest of the group, say why they are important and talk about the memories they evoke.

WHAT TO DO

Introduce the activity and invite someone to start it by showing one item from their bag and sharing their memories associated with it. Encourage others to ask questions to help the person expand on their experiences. When that person has finished, invite someone else to share an item from their bag and share their memory. Continue in this fashion until everyone has talked about each of their items.

End the activity by asking each person to choose one item and state what they think it tells them about themselves. For example: photo of a son – 'He's my pride and joy'; a book – 'I love escaping to an imaginary world. It helps me relax.'

COMMENT

It is helpful to choose five items of your own to bring along to the group so you too can participate. You can then start the activity by talking briefly about one of your items. This can make it easier for anyone who is feeling a bit nervous about the activity. Do, however, make sure the items you choose for your bag respect your private life.

Also, you can, of course, shorten the time needed for the activity by reducing the number of items you ask people to bring along.

VOICES

PURPOSE

To use voice to access memories of people and reflect on past experiences.

WHAT YOU'LL NEED

No materials needed.

WHAT TO DO

State that voices are unique to individuals. Ask:

» How would you describe the sound of your own voice?

» How would you describe the voice of the person sitting on your left?

» How do voices differ in tone and pitch? For instance, they can be shrill, sexy, sharp, comforting, condescending, tired, deep or hollow.

» Do people's voices sound different depending on the person you are with or the situation you are in?

After a brief discussion, ask people to sit quietly and think about the voices of people they have known in the past. Ask them to pick out one in particular. It might be a grandparent or other relative, a colleague, a lover, a boss, a friend or a neighbour. After a moment for people to think, invite participants, in turn, to describe the voice, the person, an incident involving them and the part they played in their life.

COMMENT

Instead of getting individuals to talk about the person, you could get them to write accounts and then read them out.

THE GOOD STUFF

PURPOSE

To remind participants about the good things which have happened to them and help them keep life in perspective.

WHAT YOU'LL NEED

Pens and paper.

WHAT TO DO

Ask individuals to make a list of ten good things that have happened to them in their life with the approximate year it occurred. A typical list might include things like:

1. *Met my best friend Ron when I was ten. (1953)*

2. *I went to stay with my aunt who introduced me to bird-watching when I was twelve. It became a lifelong hobby. (1955)*

3. *Had an argument and fell out with Ron. Made me realise I was in love with him. (1964)*

4. *Married Ron. (1965)*

5. *First child, Peter, born. (1966)*

6. *Got the sack from Thornton's furniture shop, a job I hated. Got a job with our local vet, which I loved. (1972)*

7. *Had a wonderful holiday in Italy with all the family. (1976)*

And so on.

The list doesn't have to be in year order but if people start the list from childhood it makes it easier to come up with ten good things and the year. When the lists are complete, invite participants, in turn, to choose one event and tell the group about it.

COMMENT

You can have as many rounds of participants talking about their good events as you wish. If individuals can't recall the year, they might remember what age they were when it occurred. Also, at different times and in different groups, you can vary the number of good things being listed from one to as many as they can recall. You can also vary the times in life that good things happened. For example: 'Good things that happened to me when I was a teenager, in my twenties, thirties, forties...'

These are also topics you can use for participants to write about.

MEMORY IMPROVISATIONS

PURPOSE

To share memories about life experiences.

WHAT YOU'LL NEED

A whiteboard or flipchart and marker.

WHAT TO DO

Split group members up into small groups of three or four people. Write a short list of memory categories on a whiteboard or flipchart – no more than four or five topics. These might be:

» 1950s	» Childhood and schooldays	» Family disputes
» 1960s	» Early work experience	» Relationships
» 1970s	» Love and marriage	» Hobbies
» 1980s	» The middle years	» Major life events
» 1990s	» Working life	» Funny events

These topics can be changed to suit the age and backgrounds of the group members. You can also introduce many other topics.

Each subgroup chooses one topic – it doesn't matter if two groups choose the same topic – from the list and discuss their experiences of it for about ten minutes. At this point, ask each subgroup to select one event from their experiences which will form the basis of an improvisation scene they can act out. They will need to decide:

» Who plays which character

» Where it take place

» What happens in the scene

Allow a further 5–10 minutes for the subgroups to plan what they are going to do and then have them, in turn, act out the chosen scene. Ensure that each group gets applause for their production.

COMMENT

If you use the decades as topics, it is helpful to remind everyone about a few of the major events that occurred in that decade. And if participants are confident and agree, you can, of course, invite a small audience to watch the scenes being acted out.